VERA QU . .
AND AL . .N MACAUSLAN

DYSLEXIA

WHAT PARENTS OUGHT TO KNOW

REVISED EDITION

Penguin Books

PENGUIN BOOKS

Published by the Penguin Group
27 Wrights Lane, London W8 5TZ, England
Viking Penguin Inc., 40 West 23rd Street, New York, New York 10010, USA
Penguin Books Australia Ltd, Ringwood, Victoria, Australia
Penguin Books Canada Ltd, 2801 John Street, Markham, Ontario, Canada L3R 1B4
Penguin Books (NZ) Ltd, 182–190 Wairau Road, Auckland 10, New Zealand

Penguin Books Ltd, Registered Offices: Harmondsworth, Middlesex, England

First published 1986
Reprinted 1986
Revised edition 1988

Made and printed in Great Britain by
Richard Clay Ltd, Bungay, Suffolk
Filmset in Monophoto Sabon and Rockwell

Vera Quin has done research and diagnostic work at the Learning Difficulties Clinic at St Thomas' Hospital for over twelve years and has worked since 1973 as a specialist teacher in ILEA comprehensive and primary schools, and at the Cheyne Centre for Spastics. Born into a multilingual family she went to nine schools using five languages and then to Girton College, Cambridge. She has held various appointments as a researcher and translator and taught ESL and French before turning to remedial work. She is the author of various publications to do with learning difficulties, including *Reading and Spelling Difficulties: a medical approach* (1981) written with Alan MacAuslan. She remains fully committed to giving all children access to the pleasures and intellectual benefits of reading.

Dr Alan MacAuslan has been the clinical assistant at the Learning Difficulties Clinic of St Thomas' Hospital since 1968, and is also the medical member of the London South Committee for the Employment of Disabled Persons. Born in July 1921, he graduated from Cambridge in 1943 and has been in the medical profession throughout his career. From 1974 to 1982 he was an Employment Medical Adviser in the Health and Safety Executive, working as medical officer various Employment Rehabilitation and Skill Centres. He has also been actively concerned in co-operation with the Careers Service. He is the Physician Charge of Learning Difficulties (Dyslexia) Assessment Team at the Portland Hospital for Women and Children. Dr MacAuslan has written articles related learning difficulties.

Contents

CONTENTS

Part III

CONTENTS

PART I

Chapter One
Explanation of the Book

Introduction

This book has been written for parents who are worried in case their child is 'dyslexic', and also for those parents who have been told that he is and are not quite sure what the word means. The sheer volume of professional jargon spewed out after a child has been assessed for reading and spelling difficulties, or dyslexia, can be extremely confusing. Doctors, speech therapists, psychologists and teachers may all be guilty of failing to explain why they have done certain tests on a child, what these tests amount to and what the results mean. Our experience at the Learning Difficulties Clinic at St Thomas' Hospital, London (which goes back to 1968 and covers nearly two thousand children), makes us quite certain that parents must have a full understanding of the situation facing their child in order to make sensible decisions about his future. A large part of our professional lives is spent explaining, answering parents' questions and suggesting what they can do to help their child. Fortunately there is also a great deal parents can do to prevent dyslexia.

Our experience has also taught us that what the doctor and speech therapist find in a child has a direct relationship with the way a child learns and therefore how teachers teach. If the doctor and speech therapist uncover a condition that is readily correctable and the condition (or learning disability) is successfully treated, a dramatic effect on the dyslexia follows. Teachers are then able to take advantage of the improved learning potential.

So this book aims to give enough information for parents to understand what the professionals are about. It is not intended to be read as a novel is read, starting at the beginning and going straight through to the end. We think you would prefer to read those parts that seem applicable to your family. You will find headings, sub-headings, numbered sections and cross-references (in square brackets) to help you find your way. We suggest you read this first section to the end and then pick and choose whatever interests you, skip the heavy or detailed parts, glance at the summaries, enjoy what is in the stories (drawn from the children seen at the Learning Difficulties Clinic at St Thomas' Hospital, with the names changed to preserve anonymity) and refer back to various parts as and when you need to.

You will notice that we speak in several different voices: straight medical, more diffuse 'teacher' talk, the conversational idiom of people sharing ideas. The material presented also falls into three groups: some facts are well established and well known; some ideas are accepted but not completely proven; sometimes the beliefs are little more than beliefs, still being explored, possibly to be rejected later. We remain open to new ideas, but when we are certain you will find that certainty reflected in the tone of the paragraph. You will also notice that we often repeat ourselves. This is because reading and writing are immensely complex activities, dependent for success on a huge network of variables, all more or less related and connected with each other. As we consider each variable in turn, we also mention the several others most closely affected, but as seen from a slightly different angle.

The pronouns he and she will be used to refer to the child and teacher. Despite possible charges of sexism, it makes for easier reading if these references remain constant.

The meaning of 'dyslexia'

2 At one time 'dyslexia' referred to a loss of reading ability in an adult who had previously been able to read. Diseases such as strokes could produce this.

The term 'specific developmental dyslexia' referred to children who failed to learn to read in spite of adequate schooling, normal health and normal intelligence. A difference was recognized between these children and others who were backward in reading because of lack of schooling, poor intelligence or unfamiliarity with the language in which they were being taught. A formula was worked out to take into account not only the age but also the intelligence of a child, so that 'specific reading retardation' (a term synonymous with 'specific developmental dyslexia') could be precisely identified for any particular child.

In common parlance, the phrase 'specific developmental dyslexia' became shortened to 'dyslexia', perhaps because parents whose children were reading-retarded formed self-support groups and called them 'dyslexia associations'. The word has now been broadened to cover children with spelling and writing problems. Consequently any child who fails to acquire the basic literacy skills that adults expect, or fails to acquire them as fast as adults think he should, is now labelled 'dyslexic'.

Learning disabilities

3 A physical defect like clumsiness, or an illness like recurring tonsillitis, often makes the acquisition of literacy difficult for a child even when his motivation is good. During the past twenty years doctors have come to recognize more and more biological causes and conditions which can produce dyslexia. Different patterns of dyslexia have been identified. All too rarely is a single cause found. More often several factors combine to produce dyslexia, with intelligence adding an important dimension.

In this sense dyslexia must be seen not as a disease but rather as a symptom. It is one of the purposes of this book to demonstrate why this is so.

Learning disorders

4 Distinct from the physically caused learning disabilities identified by the doctor, and often running in parallel with them, are the learning disorders. These are disturbances of learning due to emotional or environmental factors (for example, poverty, or the mother tongue being different from the language of instruction). Information about these disorders reaches the doctor from parents, teachers and perhaps the social services.

The assessment team

5 A great deal needs to be known about a child before he can be sensibly helped. Three sources of information are used to build up a picture of the whole child over a period of time. First, those adults in contact with the child on a day-to-day basis. Parents provide information on the home background, on how the child interacts with members of the family, and details of family activities since birth, while teachers provide information about the response to learning experiences and relations with the peer group over a period. Second, the child himself provides a view of his learning difficulties as part of his whole life and of any investigations into them. Finally, the investigative team is called in to assist. The team should consist of the doctor, for the medical aspects; the clinical psychologist, to determine intelligence and perceptual capabilities; the speech therapist, to examine language development and listening skills; and the teacher to pinpoint the extent of the scholastic failure. The investigative team led by the doctor obtains an in-depth view of the child at a specific moment in time. Think of it as an immensely detailed still from a film: the movie is provided by the parents and the teachers; the child is the subject of both the movie and the still, and the commentator and critic of both.

All three – parents, child and assessment team – are necessary to investigate the dyslexia. But with luck, and after reading this book, the majority of parents should avoid having to worry about learning difficulties in their children.

Summary (2–5)

6 *Dyslexia is a symptom, the cause or causes of which have to be determined before help can be given.*

The causes of dyslexia can be either biological or environmental, and often the two run in parallel.

If a child who is failing in school is to be adequately helped, the first essential is a proper investigation by a multidisciplinary team, together with consideration of his environment and his day-to-day behaviour.

Development and how it is assessed

7 If a parent or teacher notices that a child is having difficulty with learning, the first step towards helping him is to find out precisely what his difficulty amounts to. The question is not 'Is it because he never pays attention that he doesn't read as well as he should?', but 'How does he read and how much can he read?'. The aim is to document the child's actual attainments, to establish his base line.

This is where tests come in. Doctors, psychologists, therapists and teachers have a considerable number of tests at their disposal, most of them thoroughly reliable, each one aiming to investigate a particular area of functioning, often something as closely defined as the child's ability to balance when standing on one foot with eyes closed. The doctors, using medical tests, will investigate the biological functioning of the child; the psychological functioning is the province of the psychologist and speech therapist; teachers will use scholastic tests. Your child will be described to you in terms of test performance first, and you, the parent, will fit that view into the context of his performance in daily living over a period of time.

The results of the tests will be expressed in two ways: a report by the investigator, which parents would do well to read first, and a figure or a series of figures. The figure could stand for age, a quotient, a percentile or an age band.

Test age

8 Child development is pretty well documented. Anyone with access to a public library can find out at what age the average child is expected to sit up, say three-word sentences and write his name correctly. It is also possible to discover the band of normality for a particular landmark: nobody – that is, no professional (parents are different) – will get excited if a child starts using three-word sentences as early as the eighteenth month, or as late as the thirty-sixth. Both are within the norm. Incidentally, for testing purposes a child's age is given in years and completed months, so a child of 9 years, 1 month and 17 days is 9 years and 1 month old, sometimes written as C A (for chronological age) 9-01.

At any given chronological age one child's development and attainments can be compared with those of children of the same age living in the same country. These norms vary from one country to another, but for the most part in English-speaking countries the differences represent fine tuning rather than anything more substantial.

If your child is aged 9 years and 1 month and is said to manage the spelling of single words with a spelling age of 8, it means that his command of spelling is equal to that of the average 8-year-old. Just as often you may be told that his spelling quotient is 90, meaning that the average spelling quotient for a child aged 9 years and 1 month is represented by the figure 100, and your child is 10 points behind the average. You could also be told – a different way of looking at it – that your child is at the forty-fifth percentile (written thus: %45), which means that 55 per cent of all children aged 9 years and 1 month are better at spelling than he is. Or the age band given might be 7 years and 6 months to 9, showing that your child's spelling performance falls within the normal range. But in all three cases your son will have written exactly the same words correctly and made the same number of mistakes, in a total of X words.

Normative tests

So, to establish the level of a child's functioning, normative tests are used. These will show how far ahead of, or behind, the national average your child's attainments in particular areas are. These tests are designed to indicate his level of development. **9**

But normative tests yield even more useful information. The report that accompanies the test figures should give a detailed analysis of the responses the child has given. To return to spelling, as in the example above, there should be a detailed 'miscue analysis'. This will group spelling mistakes by type: for instance, has the child left out audible consonants, and if so which ones; or has he spelt correctly no more than the first two letters of each word? The detailed analysis will suggest the next questions to be asked. If the audible letters have been left out, is this a sign of hearing impairment? Consequently, what are the results of his hearing tests? If he gets no further than the first two letters of a word, which is something younger children do, is this part of a picture of general immaturity, that is, delayed development all round; or is it part of a delay with language at all levels; or a delay with literacy only, that is, with reading and spelling; or is the delay limited to spelling? In other words, the report will suggest whether the trouble is caused by delay in development, or by an unusual development.

An example will clarify this. A great many children have the interdental S, in lay language a lisp. No one is going to worry about this until the second teeth come through, for these may well provide better occlusion, and with fewer gaps the lisp should disappear. But suppose that the lisp persists to the age of ten. At this age it represents a small developmental delay. The speech therapist will, at this point, first establish whether the child lisps on all S sounds, or only if the S is the first sound, or the last, or somewhere in the middle, or if it is in combination with certain other sounds. She will investigate the possibility of an anatomical or neurological cause of the lisp, and assuming there is none she will readily bring this small backwardness to mature functioning. But imagine a child who is a clutterer. You would recognize one – and there are very few of these unusual children – by the way his speech accelerates, words become truncated and finally coherence is lost. A speech therapist faced with this picture will not delay, but immediately start investigations and corrective treatment.

In general, tests are designed for one of two functions. First, *screening*, to find out how near to the average the child is in any one area of functioning, or any related area. These tests are like a sieve. For every child that passes in every particular there is no need to worry or investigate further. And second, *diagnostic*, to examine closely the exceptional functioning, identify its causes and suggest remediation. With the last in mind, these tests are sometimes called 'diagnostic and pre-scriptive'.

In some cases, and increasingly in schools, children are assessed by criterion-referenced tests. These, as their name implies, are tests to find out how well a child is learning a particular task that is being taught over a period of time. This type of test is also used for areas of functioning that are not readily quantifiable, including socially useful tasks like tying shoelaces or packing a suitcase. In schools, handwriting is commonly assessed in this way.

Groups of tests – why they are necessary

10

Processes as complicated as reading, writing and spelling are built up from a number of related functions. Therefore, even in school, no single test will be adequate as a screen for literacy attainment. Consequently, starting with teachers in schools, test batteries – that is, a series of related tests – will be used at every stage to establish the level of functioning. For diagnostic purposes the number of tests available is obviously very considerable.

There are few illnesses which cause learning difficulties all by themselves and fewer which, if cured, are associated with complete relief of the difficulty. It is commoner to find that several factors combine to produce learning problems. Failure to recognize the importance of more than one factor can lead adults, especially professionals, to ride their own hobby horse and fail to take all the steps necessary to help the child. When weighing up the medical, or, if you prefer the term, biological, causes underlying a dyslexia, do not forget that the child's development of language, together with his level of intelligence, are of vital importance in the equation.

Some diseases cause as much trouble with their after-effects as they do when they are active. Scarring may be more difficult to deal with than the cause of the scarring and it may last much longer. Most diseases have a general as well as a local effect, though the main attention of the sufferer is focused on the part most obviously afflicted. A boil on your finger stops you using that hand, but it also makes the rest of you feel rotten. The same applies to illnesses associated with learning difficulties. There are those illnesses which affect the unborn child in the womb but which are no longer active after birth, though their damage remains. There are other diseases which cause brief, immediate problems to the infant or schoolchild but which result in substantial difficulties or delays in language development. And there are those which have a direct effect on school performance.

Chapter Two
Do You Know This Child?

Finding your way about this book

11 For those parents who recognize that they and their child have a problem but do not know where to start, we have drawn little word-pictures of different types of children with learning difficulties. The numbers of the relevant sections are given below each description. Obviously these sketches do not cover the whole range of difficulties which may be encountered, but we hope that they will lead you into the book and help you to find your way to the parts that deal with your particular problem.

Always on the go

12 Right from the time he was born, he has been impossible. He was active as a tiny and he is worse now. It is not his reading and writing so much as his behaviour in class which is the worry. He will not sit still; he disturbs the other children and is always wandering about when he should be sitting down. He is dangerous out in the street. He will walk straight across the road without any regard for the traffic. We have had to pull him back from certain death a number of times and now we dare not let him out on his own. We are all worn out, except him.

See **134** – Hyperkinesis

He never pays attention to what I say

13 The family is waiting to go out to something special, and it is time to get spruced up. 'Johnny, go upstairs, wash your hands and face, brush your hair, get a clean hanky and come down here again – quick now.' Twenty minutes later, no Johnny. 'Where is that boy?' Father fuming, mother fussing and Johnny playing with his Lego on the floor of his room; which is as far as he had got before he failed to remember what he had come upstairs for. It is worse at school. He never pays attention and is always asking the teacher to repeat what she has said. If there is homework, he has to ask some other child what he is supposed to be doing.

See 27 – Partial hearing loss
    32 – Glue ears

The clumsy kid

14

If there is a crash in the house, it's him. Ever since he was tiny he has been covered in bruises and sticking plaster. If he can knock it over, spill it or bang into it, then he will. He was cheerful until he went to school. There he had difficulty learning his letters. He does not like jig-saw puzzles and those toys where he has to build a horse or a bus out of flat bits. He is behind with reading and his spelling is bad. We never give him a boiled egg for breakfast, he gets it all down his tee-shirt and you can't send him to school like that.

See 81 – Clumsiness
    82 – Causes of clumsiness

Can't spell but can read

15

He reads reasonably well, even doing it for fun sometimes, and he reads best to himself. Reading out loud is difficult; he is slow and finds it a bit of a bore. His spelling is *awful*. He makes silly mistakes, writing out words the way they sound and not the way they should be spelt. He is always coming back from school with a number of words to learn by the next day and he has been instructed to write them out several times. He knows them immediately after he has learnt them, but has forgotten them next week. It is odd, but he may misspell a word in one line and get it right in the next. His sums may be wrong, too; he knows how to do them, but often gets the wrong answer because he puts the numbers down in the wrong order. His compositions are short and covered in crossings-out. His bad handwriting helps to disguise his worse spelling. Trying to teach him to spell at home is hopeless, everybody ends up cross. Why can't he learn to spell? Surely he could do better if only he would try.

See **72, 73** – Short-term memories

102 – I T P A visual sequential memory sub-test

He switches off

16 He was fine at the day-nursery. In fact he was fine at the infant school. The trouble began when he was about seven or perhaps a bit later. He started to 'switch off'; just not paying attention when in class. It doesn't seem to worry him. He just asks what you've said and goes on doing what he should. The trouble is that he is falling behind at school. We see him switch off occasionally. He does it more often when he's tired. Yes, he still wets the bed sometimes, even if we have woken him up and potted him before we go to bed. I think he does it in the morning. We have tried one of those alarms, but it didn't help. Granny says not to worry, he's just like one of his uncles. She says he will grow out of it.

See **120** – Epilepsy

I can't get him to school in the morning

17 Every morning it is the same, during term-time, anyway. First he won't get up because he says he feels ill. Then he is slow to dress and we are always late. Then I have to drag him down the street – I don't know what the neighbours think. When we get to the school, he won't go in and four of us have to carry him into the classroom. I wish his father was there to help. Yes, sometimes he runs home at dinner-time, but his teachers are very good and they know to watch out for this.

See **127** – Sources of stress

128 – Some stress effects

He says he can't see

18 He says he can't see and he is always complaining of headaches. We took him to have his eyes tested, but apparently he doesn't need glasses. When he reads he makes silly mistakes. The trouble is that he knows he is behind – difficult for him not to, because he is having remedial help at school. The teacher says he needs lots of phonics, but he has had that and it has not made any difference. He always reads with his head on his arm. We've warned him it will ruin his eyes if he goes on like that but he won't stop doing it.

See **44** – Patterns of print

It's the best school in the neighbourhood
19

He got on fine at first. He can read quite well, or rather we thought he could, but the school says he is behind the rest of his class. His spelling is not too bad, but he is having difficulty writing essays and his maths are weak. The school says he should stay down at the end of the year and repeat the work again. He will miss his friends when they move up and he does not. The school has suggested that he has extra help. It is beginning to worry him and his eczema has come back.

See **67** – WISC-R: a general view

He plays with younger children
20

He was late to talk. They said they were worried about him at his nursery school. Now he likes to play with younger children – I think it's because his own age group ignores him. He is a bit silent because he is shy, but he always understands what we say to him. No, he has never had any ear trouble. He likes doing things with his hands. He is very good at changing electric plugs and things. He is a nice boy. We are sure he is not stupid. He is reading simple books and his spelling is very bad.

See **90** – Vocabulary

The normal child
21

Though different children grow and develop at different rates and the boundaries of what is normal are wide, there are stages in a child's development which it is important to recognize.

Should you fear that there is a delay in his doing something by the time suggested, it is right to seek the advice of your family doctor or the child development clinic. Delay in achievement does not necessarily spell disaster, but it is as well to have some idea of what you can expect your child to do, and when. The same applies to growth. Height, weight and head circumference should be measured regularly by the clinic or the doctor. What matters is not the isolated measurement but the rate of increase in size determined over a long time. It is up to the professionals to keep an eye on the child's progress and up to the parents to take him regularly for his check-ups.

By four months, your baby should be excited when he sees his food approaching, he should like to be helped to sit upright and if you put a toy into his hand he will play with it. He should laugh. He should turn his head towards a noise.

By six months, he should sit supported in a high-chair and if you stand him up he will bounce energetically. He can kick with one foot and can roll over. He looks everywhere and squinting is no longer normal. If he drops a toy he will probably look to see where it has gone. He laughs, chuckles and squeals. Everything goes into his mouth.

By a year, he can sit for a long time; he can crawl on all fours and if you hold one hand he will walk. He should have stopped putting everything into his mouth by way of investigation, but he will be stretching out to pick up anything small which catches his eye. If he drops something, he should certainly be looking to see where it has gone. He will shout if he wants you and if he does not hear you coming he will shout again. He understands 'no-no' and will play peek-a-boo. He should know his own name. When you are dressing him, he will hold out his hand for the sleeve and his foot for the shoe. He is but a month away from walking on his own.

The two-year-old is mobile. He can run, stopping and starting with ease. He climbs up the furniture and usually does not have to be helped down again. He can go up and down stairs, two feet to each step. He dresses himself, or at least he thinks he can. If you are able to count them, he uses about fifty words; he talks incessantly and refers to himself by name. You can usually get him to join with you in nursery rhymes. Most important, he should be able to join two or three words together spontaneously. He should be dry most days, but probably will not be dry at night.

The three-year-old runs round obstacles for the fun of it. He rides a tricycle. He walks upstairs like an adult, but still comes down two feet to a step. He can certainly dress himself, except for those very difficult buttons. He should be dry at night. If you give him a pencil he will make a shot at copying a circle. He talks away to himself still and has begun to ask questions. He is more or less tidy. He is loving.

The four-year-old goes up and down stairs like an adult. He can run on tip-toe and skip or hop. He can stand on one foot. He can manage in the toilet. He is cheeky, is always asking questions and is beginning to do what he wants rather than what you want. He will listen to long stories and will tell you some of his own in return. He likes to play with other children, and is sometimes bossy and sometimes helpful with them. He should be able to copy a cross and probably the letters V, H, T and O. He can draw a person with head and legs and usually knows three or four colours.

The five-year-old is an active show-off, skipping, sliding, swinging and even perhaps dancing to music. Much less cheeky and much more sensible, he has a fine independence in familiar surroundings. He has his own friends and will play well with them. He can repeat four numbers, count the fingers of one hand and should be able to name four colours. He can copy a square and a triangle and may be able to write a few letters on his own.

This index of activities is brief: different aspects of a child's development are discussed in much greater detail in other sections of the book. The expanding capabilities which take place during normal growth are listed alongside descriptions of what can go wrong so that parents may recognize when help should be sought. The contrast between what should happen and what should not is drawn in a variety of fields.

Patterns of normal development in these fields are detailed in the following sections:

PART II

Introduction

In Part II you will find details of how the body systems work towards **22** reading and spelling, and how things can go wrong. The chapters have been arranged so that the receptor, or sensory, systems (which gather information from the world around us) come first. Common diseases which affect these systems and therefore have an impact on reading and spelling are included in the appropriate chapters. Then come details of the brain's anatomy and functioning, which show how it deals with the incoming information. The difference between the brain of a child and that of an adult is emphasized. There is some discussion on the development of the one into the other. Perception, intelligence, memory and language follow and then an outline of those factors which can have an effect on brain function. Finally there is a brief résumé of the current position on specific developmental dyslexia, hyperkinesis and minimal cerebral dysfunction.

The whole is a hotch-potch or medley of medical factors which have either been suspected of causing dyslexia or have been proved to do so. They have been included because cases have been seen in the authors' clinic, or because parents have raised questions on particular topics.

The admonitions and advice which run through Part II have all been promoted, at one time or another, by problems confronting parents. We have tried to bring our clinic experience to bear on what we have been writing. So if you feel that the obvious has been stated, please remember that once, at least, it wasn't clear to someone else.

Very few medical conditions are directly related to learning disabilities in the sense that if the disease is cured then the dyslexia vanishes. More commonly the illness combines with other factors, such as a low IQ or emotional disturbance, to produce either a general or a specific learning difficulty. In such cases, curing the illness makes a difference but is not the only answer.

There are some diseases and injuries which, when severe, cause damage to the brain and reduce the ability to learn and develop normally. When the same conditions are mild, the results may also be mild. The probability of a gradient of disaster running from death through severe damage, moderate damage, mild damage and finally no damage at all has been suggested in much of the literature about dyslexia. Put simply, if severe trauma produces cerebral palsy with marked visuo-perceptual problems, may not mild trauma result in spelling problems without any physical disability?

The Japanese experience at Minnemata is a good example of this and we retail it here to illustrate the gradation of disease which may occur, though there is practically no likelihood of a similar disaster occurring in the United Kingdom. In Japan, methyl mercury was discharged from a plastics factory into the sea; the chemical became concentrated in fish which were then eaten by the local people. A high proportion of children born in the following years had cerebral palsy, though some of the mothers were quite unaffected. Then a significant number of the children who appeared to have escaped early damage were found to have problems of coordination. The methyl mercury absorbed by the child while in his mother's womb was capable of being responsible for six Ds: birth deficits, abnormal development, deviant behaviour, neurological disorder, immunological deficiencies and death. It seems that if a lot of something does you a lot of damage, then a little of it may do you a small amount of harm.

Chapter Three
Hearing

A recent survey estimated that twenty-nine per cent of children with **23** learning difficulties in the Inner London area had significant histories of ear disease. The importance of ear disease as a cause of poor language development and hence poor reading cannot be too strongly stressed, especially as cure and therefore prevention of the learning disability is possible.

The measurement of noise

Sound is energy; the greater the physical effort put into shouting, the **24** louder the shout. Loudness is measured in decibels. The scale is logarithmic, which means that ten decibels are ten times louder than one decibel, but that twenty decibels are a hundred times louder than one, and thirty decibels a thousand times louder.

Sound travels in waves of different frequencies. The higher the noise the shorter are the waves, and therefore the crests of the waves occur more frequently. In normal speech, these frequencies range from 100 to 100,000 wave cycles per second. The ear is the organ which catches the sound waves, turning them into nerve impulses which are relayed to the brain for interpretation.

The ear

The ear has three parts – outer, middle and inner. Each part is separated **25** from the other by a drum. The outer ear consists of the ear flap and the ear hole, both of which are easily visible. Losing an ear flap does not greatly hinder hearing, nor does wax in the ear hole, unless the wax gets wet and swells. The ear drum at the bottom of the ear hole is much more important. It vibrates in response to the sound waves which reach it. It forms the outer wall of the middle ear as well as the inner wall of the outer ear.

Sound waves do not travel across the cavity of the middle ear by air but by the movement of three tiny bones, each of which moves the next, the last one hitting a very small inner ear drum. These little bones

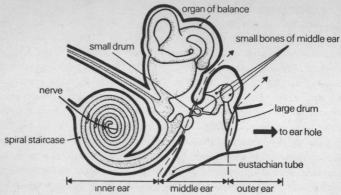

Figure 1   The middle and inner ear

are a gearing system which concentrates the energy spread across the large outer drum on to the smaller surface of the inner drum. This receives a harder 'punch', which is necessary because the inner ear is like a spiral staircase (the cochlea) filled with fluid. The 'stair carpet' is composed of nerve cells which are stimulated by the shock waves travelling through the fluid and which send nerve impulses to the brain. (See Figure 1.) Most of the waves reach the fluid of the inner drum via this system, though some may travel through the bones of the head, which can also transmit sound but not so effectively.

For the outer drum to work efficiently, the pressures on each side of it must be equal. The air pressure in the atmosphere and the air pressure in the middle ear must be the same, or the drum will be distorted and will not vibrate properly. This happens when we fly or go up a mountain. At a height, atmospheric pressure is less than in the valley below, so the pressure on the outside of the drum becomes lower than that in the middle air. To balance the two, some air escapes down the Eustachian tube (which runs from the middle ear to the back of the nose), like bath water running down the overflow pipe.

Testing hearing

26 There are two simple hearing tests which are a necessary part of any diagnostic programme for the identification of causes of learning disabilities. Both must be carried out, since one test only can lead to misleading views of a patient's hearing ability. Both should be done by a qualified tester, preferably an audiometrist.

Pure tone audiometry

This tests a child's ability to hear sounds of different frequencies. The test should be carried out in a soundproof booth. If none is available, then any suspicious negative results must be checked using such a booth. Suspicious positive results will be followed up as a matter of course. Through properly fitting headphones, the child hears sounds of different frequencies. Each sound, presented as though it came from a distance of six feet from the child, is made softer and softer until the patient can no longer hear it. The tester does not sit in the booth, but she and the child can see one another. The child has to press a button every time he hears the sound. The results are shown on a graph and indicate the number of decibels required for a sound of a given frequency to be just audible. Bone as well as air conduction of sound may be tested.

Parents faced with the results must appreciate two points. First, the degree of hearing loss relates to the average amount of noise which an average person can hear at six feet. Second, slight hearing loss, whether in one ear or both, is of greater significance to the child developing language than to the child or adult who has already done so. Pure tone audiometry is sometimes combined with electro-encephalography to distinguish between genuine hearing loss and that due to emotional causes.

The impedance bridge test or tympanography

To find out what the air pressure in the middle ear may be, a soft probe is placed in the child's outer ear and the ear hole is gently sealed off. A quiet sound is 'bounced' off the ear drum back to the probe. At the same time, the pressure in the outer ear may be slightly altered. When the pressure in the middle ear equals that in the outer ear, then the amount of energy reflected back to the probe is least, most of it going on across the middle ear to stimulate the nerves in the inner ear. The equal pressures enable the drum to vibrate properly. If there is fluid in the middle ear, then the vibrations of the drum are reduced, more sound energy is reflected back to the probe and less gets across to the inner ear.

The whole business of inserting the probe and testing takes about five minutes. It is painless and does not require the child to say what he hears but only to sit still and quiet. The results come out as a curve, with the air pressure in the outer ear canal along the horizontal axis of a graph and the 'compliance' (amount of movement of the drum) along the vertical axis. If there is an alteration in compliance with alterations

35

of the pressure in the outer ear, the result is a flattish curve which suggests that fluid in the middle ear is stopping the drum from vibrating normally. If the compliance peaks when there is a negative pressure in the outer ear relevant to the atmospheric pressure, this suggests a negative pressure in the middle ear, indicating blocking of the Eustachian tube, as may occur with catarrh.

Partial hearing loss

27 The term 'partial hearing loss' covers several different conditions. It can imply a general reduction to hear all frequencies, or a selective reduction in hearing ability for some frequencies, or hearing reduction in one ear only.

The significance of a general reduction in the ability to hear depends not only on the degree of loss, but also on the time of onset in relation to a child's stage of language development, on the intelligence of the child, on the richness of the family's language environment and on the speed with which the condition is recognized.

The different noises which make up speech are produced with different degrees of loudness depending on what they are. Vowels are said more loudly than consonants. Different speech sounds fall into different frequency bands; vowels are in the lower and middle frequencies, consonants in the middle and higher ones. To hear accurately what someone else is saying, we require not only good overall hearing but also good hearing in all frequencies. A loss of forty decibels or more in both ears has a significant effect on a child's language development. There is some doubt about the importance of slighter losses. The other factors mentioned above are very relevant in such cases. A loss of twenty-five decibels has little effect on a child whose language is well developed, though he had better not sit at the back of the class. But the same loss can produce reduced listening skills [73], poor processing of auditory material [98] and poor speech sound discrimination in a younger or less bright child.

Selective reduction affecting certain frequencies is important. A high-tone hearing loss reduces the ability to hear some consonants and produces the same effect as being at a noisy party when you cannot quite hear what is being said. It causes distress and frustration to the young child, with all the usual upsets of bad behaviour, stomach-aches, headaches and poor reading and spelling which go hand-in-hand with not being able to understand what is being said in class.

A case in point serves to illustrate what happens if such selective reduction in hearing goes unrecognized.

Olivia came to the clinic when she was twenty-three. Pretty, shy and self-deprecating, she had been urged to seek help by her boyfriend, who had found it embarrassing when she did not answer when spoken to. She was fed up with her menial job in the linen room of a hospital, mending torn pillowcases and sheets all day. She had hoped to take a special needlework qualification, but because she could not read she was unable to pass the necessary qualifying exams or read the set books. She had been educated abroad until the age of ten, because her father worked overseas; she then came back to England and attended a boarding school as her parents remained abroad. She was thought to be unintelligent, almost educationally subnormal, but as she was sweet, biddable and caused no problems she was allowed to drift along, going at her own pace as a slow learner. She left school with no academic qualifications but was skilful with a needle.

Investigation showed that she had a severe high-tone hearing loss. She had a reading age of eight and could barely spell. She had picked up lipreading and was proficient at it, so proficient that her language and communication were excellent, provided that she could see who she was speaking to. She was given hearing aids and registered as disabled, and the college where she wished to train was told of her disability and accepted her. Special provision at examination times was arranged. Recognized as deaf by society, official and unofficial attitudes changed towards her. With luck, she will achieve her qualification and go on to work which will satisfy her potential. But what a wasted life to date, and what a reflection on a system that could condemn without investigation.

One-sided hearing loss

One-sided, or unilateral, hearing loss is a deceptive condition. If an adult is a bit deaf in one ear, it only causes a little irritation: 'Sit on my other side, I can hear better if you do.' For the child whose language and reading skills are well developed, the problems are much like those of the adult. Sitting on the wrong side of the classroom with the bad ear towards the teacher will make it difficult to hear what is said and easy to become inattentive. For a younger child, a unilateral hearing loss

28

may be assumed to be unimportant: 'He can hear perfectly well with his left ear and he always answers when I speak to him, so why doesn't he learn to read?'

There are two ways of learning to read, using opposite halves of the brain [57]. The right half deals with what is seen, what is perceived visually, so that the shape of the word is recognized. The left half deals with speech and the sounds of speech. The functions of the two halves should combine to produce accurate, fluent reading.

Sounds are heard by both sides of the brain. Most impulses from one ear cross to the opposite side, so that the left ear supplies the right half of the brain and vice versa. In the same way that some of us are right- and some left-handed, we are also right- or left-eared [60]. A hearing loss in the dominant ear, coming between the firm establishment of that dominance and the commencement of learning to read, may have an effect on the early acquisition of reading skills. Partial deafness of one ear can make learning to read difficult.

Spotting the partially hearing child

29 A normal child with normal hearing should develop normal listening, normal speech and normal language. Listening is paying attention to what people say and to all other sounds; speech is talking normally and making the correct word sounds; and language is the turning of thoughts into sounds so that others know what you mean.

Before parents can hope to spot that something is amiss with their child's hearing, they must have some idea of the normal rate of development of listening, speech and language. This is discussed fully under 'Language' in Chapter 9, but here is a quick guide. Do please remember that it is only a rough one.

Just after his first birthday, you should recognize some words among your child's babblings. A few months later he will begin to understand some simple commands and act upon them. By eighteen months, he will enjoy nursery rhymes and he will probably join in in an inefficient way. He will point to familiar things if you encourage him to do so. He lets you know what he wants by pointing at an object and will perhaps add a word or two to back up his demands.

The two-year-old chatters to himself while he plays and he begins to have make-believe games. Sentences – small ones, it is true – should be formed by two and a half, but words are definitely strung together with meaning. He enjoys being read to and will say simple nursery rhymes for you.

By three, he has discovered 'Why?'. He is easy to understand, though he still uses some baby-talk. Most of this should have gone by the time he is four, when he will listen to quite long stories and tell rambling ones of his own. If you use a new word he will ask what it means.

So what about the partially deaf child? He does not pass the milestones at the same time as he should. But variations within normality are wide. As a general rule, you should seek advice if:

– your tiny baby does not respond to sounds by turning towards them;
– your slightly bigger baby does not imitate noises made by you;
– your child does not make sentences by the age of three;
– he has not abandoned baby-talk by the age of four.

If your child is not talking at all by the time he is three, the situation is urgent.

Causes of deafness

There are a large number of diseases which can cause deafness or **30** partial deafness. A lot of them are avoidable. The normal medical surveillance extended to mother and baby before and during the birth guard against most of the conditions that threaten hearing. During childhood, certain illnesses can affect hearing subtly and pass almost unnoticed until the child gets to school and fails to learn to read and spell. By far the most important of these are infections of the middle ear, which account for almost thirty per cent of learning disabilities among children.

Brief accounts of the following five medical conditions are given so that parents can be on their guard and ask for help should they suspect that one or other of the illnesses is having an effect on their child's language development or school performance: infections of the middle ear in early life; glue ears; nerve deafness; central hearing loss; and mouth-breathing.

Infections of the middle ear in early life

If the Eustachian tube (see Figure 1, p. 34) becomes temporarily blocked, **31** we are a bit deaf and slightly uncomfortable. If, however, it becomes blocked as the result of a cold in the nose and that infection goes up the tube into the middle ear, then inflammation sets in. Pus forms behind the drum and we get ear-ache. In a small child, the immediate result is pain – the child is fretful, feverish and crying. No amount of feeding, cuddling or walking him about the room in your arms makes any difference. The doctor is called and in the course of his examination he will look down the ears. If he sees signs of middle-ear disease, he may prescribe an antibiotic; relief comes in a matter of hours. When the pain, fever and distress have subsided, the medicine may well be stopped by the parents. But, though the pain has gone, the Eustachian tube may still be blocked and some fluid may persist in the middle ear for up to four months in a few cases. (Not the 'glue ears' described in 32.)

The child may be partially deaf because of impairment of the outer drums' function, for as much as three months after each attack of ear-ache. During this time the child will find it difficult to hear precisely what his mother is saying. He may find it easier to busy himself with his own thoughts rather than respond to the half-heard world outside. The impact on his language skills will be shortlived, but the effect on his listening skills may be marked. Five or more attacks of acute middle-ear infection, requiring medical treatment, before a child is six years old may be enough to retard his ability to remember what is said immediately after he has heard it.

Such children come to school with well-developed language, that is good vocabularies, normal expressive language and syntax up to their age level [90, 91, 94], but they never seem to pay attention and never do what they are told. You can tell such a child to go upstairs, wash his hands, put on clean socks, get a clean hanky, brush his hair and come down again. He goes upstairs but nothing happens when he gets there. You tell him something and five minutes later he has forgotten it. He must be deaf. His hearing is checked. It is normal (but it wasn't when he was younger). He is not deaf so he must be naughty, but he isn't.

What has happened is that his listening ability and his memory for what has been said have not developed properly. He can only hear and digest a limited number of sounds at any one time. Give him a long series of commands without pause and he is lost. All the noise information in so short a time is too much for him to absorb. He has lost all except the very first and last bits of what you have said. Given information in smaller chunks with pauses in between sentences, where full stops and commas might be if it was written, he can cope. Give him instructions in gobbets so that he can take them on board. It takes time to improve matters, but if you understand the problem and realize that it rests in the way in which adults present information to him, that is half the battle. Think of the same child in the school situation. The teacher is strange, other children are distracting, the subject matter is new. The lesson may be long. Before it is half over the child is lost, missing the point of the lesson and learning nothing. Soon he shifts from being a poor listener to being a poor understander. But his chances of being a good reader are the same as a child who has not had middle-ear disease. He should score well on the weekly single word spelling test, but ask him to write a dictated passage of continuous prose [173] and the result is a disaster. Preventative action is best. If your child has five or more attacks of middle-ear disease before he is six, ask your doctor to refer him to a speech therapist. She will tell you if there has been a hold-up in the development of listening skill. If there has been, she will tell you how it can be improved. She may advise parents and teachers what to do, what games to play and how bad the problem really is.

If the child is already at school, it helps if the therapist and the teacher get together to work out the best way of helping the child. It is unlikely that the therapist will need to give him therapy sessions. At the same time, it is important to get his hearing checked to make sure there is no persisting deafness. If attacks of ear-ache persist, seek medical advice.

The first thing that went wrong for David was an accute attack of ear-ache when he was two years old. From then on he had two or three attacks a year, usually when he caught a cold, until he was six. At one time the doctor got fed up with being called out at all hours to see him, so a bottle of antibiotic syrup was kept in the refrigerator for use when the ear-ache started.

By the time he was six, he was difficult to understand. He spoke far too quickly and his words were slurred one into the other. His parents could understand his jargon, but no one else could. He was given speech therapy and he became much easier to understand.

However, he had, according to the therapist, poor listening skills. When the doctor at the clinic asked him to 'slip off your shirt and trousers but leave on your underpants and jump on to the couch so that I can see how strong you are', nothing happened. He stood in the examination room fiddling with a button and then began to play with the blood pressure machine on the table. The requests were re-phrased in simple chunks 'Take off your trousers' – so he did. 'Take off your shirt' – success. 'Jump up here' – and he was on the couch in a flash. His understanding of what was said to him was dependent on the number of sounds he had to take in. His auditory sequential memory was very poor [73].

This defect had a minimal effect at home where he knew what was going on or likely to happen, but was of great importance in the classroom situation where all the messages were unfamiliar and the verbal output of the teacher long. There was never any chance of his asking for a repeat.

To refurbish his listening skills, lost during the intermittent patches of partial deafness after each attack of middle-ear disease, the adults dealing with him were asked to 'chunk' their requests to him. They were encouraged to pause when speaking, at those places where there would be a punctuation mark if the message had been a written one.

The speech therapist visited the school and suggested various ideas which could be incorporated into the curriculum to encourage listening. For example, she recommended that, at the beginning of the day, the class should be told that somewhere in the lesson the teacher would say a particular word. The children were told to listen out for this word and the first person to hear it would be given a reward.

Summary (31)

If your child has had five or more attacks of bad ear-ache before the age of six, get a speech therapist to see him.

If he has had five or more attacks of ear-ache but is now at school and inattentive, still get the speech therapist to see him.

If he has poor listening skills, she will tell you, and probably his teacher, how he can be helped.

Glue ears

32 What does the expression 'glue ears' mean?

The Eustachian tube (see Figure 1, p. 34) becomes blocked; the cells lining the middle ear secrete a mucus which cannot drain away down the tube, and the mucus thickens to a sticky glue. This works like the soft pedal of a piano, damping down the vibrations of the outer drum and slowing the transmission of sounds. The child becomes partially deaf. Every time he catches a cold, he may get ear-ache; a child may complain that his 'head rattles every time I shake it'. This is understandable if he has just come out of a swimming pool, but not at other times. If he has a cleft palate, glue ear is a common complication. During the times of ear-ache, he will suffer in the same way as the child with repeated attacks of ear-ache. But, in addition to having poor listening skills, he may not acquire the recognition of speech sounds at the usual time. A lot depends on when the glue develops: the earlier this happens, the more troublesome it can be. If the condition starts before seven, he may have marked difficulty with speech sound discrimination by the time he gets to school. He may find it difficult to know whether someone has said 'bin' or 'pin' [93].

Sound blends, such as 'ft' or 'ng', may be hard for him to distinguish. Both these problems will lead to a reduction in his receptive vocabulary (that is, the number of words he understands), some difficulty with general comprehension, and a positive loss of what is being said in class.

A simple 'sweep' audiological screening test may not pick up his problem. This may reinforce a teacher's view that he is a naughty little boy who does not listen. At home, his problems will not be so noticeable. Families do and say the same things at about the same time each day, children vanish upstairs and play by themselves, there is much one-to-one talking, and body language is well understood.

If glue ears are suspected, a tympanogram [26] as well as a pure tone audiogram must be done. If the ear, nose and throat specialist confirms the diagnosis, he will drain the ears. This may be done simply by prescribing appropriate nose drops to open up the Eustachian tube, or it may be necessary to drain the ears and insert grommets to ensure that the glue does not re-accumulate.

When the glue ears are cured, it still remains to correct any residual loss of language or listening skills. This can be harder than the drainage procedure. The speech therapist must be consulted and she will decide what needs to be done, if anything. Her findings and recommendations must be passed on to parents and teachers. Lost ground has to be made up before the child can be expected to realize his potential.

The language and listening skills improve rapidly, and reading achievement should pick up hand-in-hand with them. Unfortunately, spelling may well be seriously affected, perhaps because the child has abandoned left cerebral hemisphere strategies [57] and has no good sound/symbol coding system on which to rely.

Henry was referred to the clinic by the eye specialist who had corrected a squint, and had been asked if there was any

connection between Henry's poor school performance and his eye condition. The situation had been made acute by Henry's form teacher, who had said that she thought he was educationally subnormal and needed special schooling. He had a past medical history of many attacks of tonsillitis but had never had middle-ear disease. He was a happy, outgoing lad, with lots of friends but a reputation for not concentrating in the classroom.

The speech therapist found that he had a very poor auditory sequential memory [73] and that his understanding of what was said to him was diminished as a result. He could not understand sound blends and his attempt to reproduce them was poor [92]. He could not read and he could not spell. He had word boundary [162], did not know what a rhyme was but could write his own name. His sums and number work were good.

The pure tone audiogram [26] showed that he had a bilateral hearing loss of fifty decibels in most frequencies. The cause was glue. His ears were drained. Eight months after the operation he came back to the clinic again, reading at his age level, lively and still happy, but though his spelling had improved this was still not his strong point.

Summary (32)
Glue ears means fluid behind the drum.
It makes the child hard of hearing.
It slows language development.
Pure tone audiometry is not enough; tympanography must be carried out too in order to make the diagnosis.
Draining the glue relieves the mechanical condition.
Speech therapy is needed to catch up lost time.
Spelling is often considerably affected even after treatment.

Nerve deafness

33 A partial loss of hearing may result from damage to the 'spiral staircase' of the inner ear (see Figure 1, p. 34) or from damage to the auditory nerve leading to the mid-brain. There may be a general reduction in hearing or a specific loss of hearing in some frequencies. Nerve deafness is the usual cause of a high-tone hearing loss. The clinical picture which results from nerve deafness is similar to that produced by middle-ear disease, but of course the story of past events will be different. The cause may be difficult to identify if the damaging disease has been forgotten or was not recorded. There may be a history of the mother having suffered a virus infection during her pregnancy, or else some trauma or infection affecting the child just prior to the loss of hearing.

The amount of language delay is dependent on the age of the child at the time of onset, and his intelligence level is very relevant. Diagnosis is in the hands of the specialist and therefore the child must be referred for an opinion. Treatment depends on what is found.

The head teacher, who had known Anna since the infants class, suggested that she should come to the clinic. It seemed that in school (which had a reputation for high standards and excellent music) Anna had no friends, was aggressive and conscious of not doing well. Her mother explained that Anna refused to communicate with her. The poor lady was puzzled why Anna should continue to have a fiercely selective memory and be bottom of the class, when her eyes had been tested, glasses for TV and school prescribed and conscientiously worn. Anna, aged just eleven, was sweet, with a charming smile and nails bitten to the quick. Yes, she did play the piano, the recorder and the guitar a bit, but it wasn't fun; yes, maths was easy (confirmed by school) but reading was a bore, writing stories hard, single-word 'spellings' easy, dictations dire. She liked drawing and riding her bike; the prospect of six more years of school with more and more reading and writing was very gloomy.

When tested, her reading accuracy was about six months below the normal for her age (nothing much to worry about) but her understanding of what she read was way, way down. Her understanding of single words was equally poor. She had beautiful handwriting and wrote single words to dictation perfectly. But in a passage of continuous prose she left out words, left out or added audible letters, changed the number of syllables in words. Clearly she could not cope with longer passages of spoken language. The psychologist found her IQ to be average and the doctor found that she was deaf, so referral to an ENT clinic was arranged. A month later, when this appointment had not been kept, her mother was re-contacted. Oh, she hadn't understood that Anna was meant to see another doctor. Was Anna really deaf, and did it really matter? Well . . . actually . . . yes, especially as she turned out to be suffering from nerve deafness.

Central hearing loss

34 Besides partial deafness arising from damage to or disease of the ear, it is possible to suffer from a condition affecting the brain which prevents accurate reception of messages coming in from the sound receiving system. Standard testing of the ears will not show the presence of disease, but even so the child does not respond to sound. In such cases referral to an appropriate specialist for full investigation is necessary and your general practitioner is the person to guide you. There may be other things amiss – a concomitant loss of motor function [76], for example. In cases of central deafness, the provision of a hearing aid is of no value.

Testing may involve the use of both the audiogram and the electro-encephalogram [121], in combination. This can be helpful in assessing very small children, where it may be difficult to distinguish between peripheral and central hearing loss.

The partially deaf child and the telephone

35 If your child has a learning disability associated with a partial hearing loss, he may be fitted with a hearing aid to boost his auditory acuity.

Nearly thirty years ago, telephones used quite a lot of electrical current and had a strong magnetic field. This could produce a whistle in a hearing aid, so a T-switch was fitted to the aid to utilize the magnetism and eliminate the whistle. Later, new kinds of telephones were introduced and these were incompatible with hearing aids. It was not until about five years ago that a way was found round this, but the necessary gadgetry was not always fitted in public telephone booths. Now there are new types of telephones full either of microchips or crystals. These use so little electricity that the hearing aids are unable to pick up the sounds.

You can get an old-fashioned type of instrument installed in your own home, but at work a firm may be using a brand new system for internal and external communication. This may present a problem for the school-leaver who wears a hearing aid and is seeking a job. In Great Britain, the local Careers Centres have an officer who deals with the placement of disabled school leavers. It is worth going to talk to him or her about the problem.

Mouth-breathing and adenoids

Though not strictly a hearing problem mouth-breathing due to enlarged adenoids falls within the province of the same sort of specialist, so it has been included in this chapter.

When a child goes to sleep, the muscular walls at the back of the throat relax and fall inwards, so narrowing the air passage from the nose and mouth to the lungs. The adenoids lie at the back of the nose and if enlarged will obstruct the air passage, especially during sleep.

The child with enlarged adenoids sleeps badly. He may talk in his sleep, wet the bed, wake up from time to time with a snort, and he snores. If observed when asleep, he may be seen to stop breathing for short periods. If he does so at least thirty times a night his school performance will be poor. During the day he will look congested about his nose, breathe through his mouth, and be drowsy and inattentive. His reading and spelling performance declines, but there is no specific problem. Taking out the adenoids cures the child. It is necessary to check hearing at the same time in case there are blocked Eustachian tubes or glue ears. The ear, nose and throat surgeon will usually do this. Surgeons are reluctant to take out the adenoids of children over the age of ten, because they know that the adenoids will shrink with the passage of time and that the enlargement will get better spontaneously. If there is doubt about the relationship of the adenoid enlargement to school performance, it may be necessary to take the child into hospital for a short time to monitor his breathing during the night. If the condition is mild, a cure may be achieved by using decongestive nose drops. Whatever the chosen course of treatment, relieving the permanently blocked nose improves school performance.

Emily was referred to the clinic because she was falling behind with her reading and spelling, in spite of remedial help (half an hour twice a week).

Apparently she had had no trouble when she first went to school, but after the age of seven she began to lag behind the others. Now, a year before she was due to move to a comprehensive school, both her parents and her teachers had become very worried about her. The main complaint was that she was inattentive, lazy and never did anything unless prodded. She was thought not to be very bright. She had friends and she liked watching TV; when asked what she did best, she replied, 'Lie in bed in the morning.'

She was long and thin, with prominent teeth which were noticeable because her mouth was always open. Her nose was stuffed up and she did not breathe through it. She had swallowed lots of antihistamines, to no avail. She snored at night. When she had gone to camp in the holidays, all the other girls in her hut had complained about the noise she made at night. Her mother said that she could be heard 'rumbling away' in bed.

Her IQ was average; her basic literacy skills (reading and spelling) were about eighteen months below the expected age level.

An X-ray of her face revealed grossly enlarged adenoids, blocking the air passage from her nose to her windpipe; there was some fluid in her antrum (sinus).

Her adenoids were taken out: six months later she was a new girl, bouncy, uncongested and catching up on lost time.

Damage limitation

37 Preventative action is best. If your child has repeated attacks of middle-ear disease before the age of six, check that no hearing loss is present and seek medical advice if the attacks of ear-ache persist. Just as important, ask your family doctor to refer your child to the local speech therapist. She will tell you if there has been any hold-up in the development of listening skills. If there is, she will suggest how they can be improved. She may say that his language is up to scratch but that you and other adults should speak to him face to face, maintaining eye contact, for so long after each attack of the ear-ache.

She may suggest listening games: identify the source of sounds; listen for sounds that are alike or different; listen for particular words that rhyme or start with the same sound and the players have to clap when the word comes up; describe a particular toy, and the child has to identify it from the description; say nursery rhymes, but leave out words for him to fill in; say nursery rhymes to various clapping rhythms to include clapping your hands on his; 'I went shopping and I bought'; thinking of words that are, or sound alike, two words joined together, like 'lampshade'; identify the product advertised on TV from the sound-track only; invent slogans from the letters on car number-plates (for instance, BAN can be expanded into British Association of Nuisances).

A common piece of advice is that the child should be given

instructions and information in small chunks, with pauses in between. As long as his syntax and vocabulary are in order he will be able to cope well with such instructions as: 'Go upstairs' (pause), 'Wash your hands' (pause), 'Brush your hair'. Don't say, 'And don't forget to brush your hair'. That is too big a chunk. Tell him what you want him to do in gobbets of speech. You will find it all gets done. He will learn that what you say has meaning, so he will learn to listen. Given time, his listening will improve, as long as you understand his problem.

If the child is at school, it is helpful if the teacher and the speech therapist can talk together, in order to find the best way of helping the child. The teacher may give him extra practice through games to break up words into syllables and to identify initial and final sounds. She may have her own way and specific materials for teaching him letter sounds.

An older child who has not developed listening habits can't re-member the longer kind of discourse a teacher will use when teaching and a pupil should use when expressing himself in writing. The child cannot hold in mind the continuum of internal speech for as long as it takes to get it down on paper. So his 'stories' become an incoherent shambles, because he is going through successive re-inventing cycles, each one going back almost to the start. There is often a second effect: the child fails to develop verbal strategies to help him process visual information. He will not use verbal labels to distinguish between the components of something seen in 3D, or in a picture/design/map sequence. It then becomes difficult to make sense and remember what has been seen. Before long, visual stimuli may be treated in the same cursory fashion as auditory ones. Teachers find the child inattentive and super-ficial and mutter about poor motivation. Come the run-up to public examinations, the child has great trouble in organizing information derived from text, observation or diagram into coherent paragraphs, each containing one main idea developed with supporting details.

Over the years of schooling, poor listening can significantly affect a child's total cognitive development. So the course of action for a child with repeated attacks of ear-ache before the age of six is: get in touch with your family doctor, the speech therapist and perhaps the ENT surgeon.

Summary (27-37)
Ears, noses and throats that are not working properly cause a vast amount of trouble. So look out for these warning signs:
1. The child has a bunged-up nose, snores, is wakeful at night but dozy during the day;

2. *He has repeated colds or sore throats;*

3. *He does not pay attention, particularly if there is another background noise, for example T V or children talking;*

4. *He plays with children a good deal younger than himself, is slow to read and is a rotten speller;*

5. *He has repeated attacks of painful ear-ache, which get better quickly when he takes medicine.*

Request a full hearing test at a hospital, and ask to see the speech therapist. She can help a great deal. Do this as soon as possible. The later you leave it, the less can be done to improve learning.

Chapter Four
Vision

Introduction

Because reading is an extension of spoken language, hearing and sound rate higher than vision and light as possible routes to learning disabilities. But the ability to see underpins the development of language.

A firework goes up into the sky, scatters a shower of pretty stars, all the colours of the rainbow. Sighted people look up and say, 'Aaaah', while the born-blind wonder what it is all about. Colours and space beyond the reach of their hands are not part of their experience. They have no internal picture of 'star', 'pretty', 'colour', 'sky'.

The adult eye

The eye is a globe filled with jelly. Behind a curved bow-window, the cornea, is a small black hole, the pupil. It is the centre of the pigmented disc, the iris, which gives our eyes their colour. Behind the pupil is the lens; its shape can be altered by a muscle so that its focal length changes. The back wall of the globe is lined by the retina which plays the part of the film in a camera by responding to light. In the middle of the retina is a small pit, the fovea, and near it is a blind spot where the nerve fibres from the retina run towards the brain. The whole is encased in a tough skin to which are attached the muscles that move the eye in its socket. (See Figure 2.)

38

When light falls on to the cells of the retina, impulses are sent down the nerve to the back part of the brain. Before reaching the brain, half the fibres in the nerve cross over to the other side. This means that each half of the brain receives messages from both eyes.

Looking

We may be civilized now, but there is a dog beneath the skin of every one of us. Anatomically and functionally we are all primitive primates. When we were surviving on the chalk downs of Wiltshire or in the woods of the Alleghenies, our eyes had to serve two basic functions. They had to pinpoint our future dinner and at the same time keep us

39

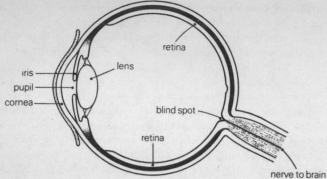

Figure 2   The eye

alert so that we did not become somebody else's mid-day meal. These two functions are still performed by our eyes.

The fovea contains a high concentration of light receptor cells. Images which fall on to it are seen more clearly than those picked up by other parts of the retina. Aim a rifle and the visual chain is 'target – foresight – backsight – middle of the lens – fovea'. Pull the trigger and the bullet should go straight to the bull. Only one eye 'takes aim'; it is called the 'dominant' eye. In right-handed people it is usually the right eye [79].

The outer area of the retina responds to movements and warns of changes in objects in the whole visual field. We may not know what has moved, but something catches our eye and we turn the head so that the fovea bears on the new object. The eyes then make rapid little movements, flickering over a target to explore all its features. These movements were first observed in people reading. Children with learning disabilities show abnormal eye movements when reading, but whether these are the cause of the dyslexia or the result is not known.

The child's eye

40 A baby's eye has some growing to do after birth. The eyeball of the newborn is only three-quarters the size of an adult one. As a result, the lens has difficulty focusing an image on to the retina. In the same way as long-sighted adults have eyeballs which are too small, so has a baby. The lens can only focus the image behind the retina and not sharply on to it. So a baby sees things a bit blurred – but does not realize this, of course. At the same time, neither the retina nor the fovea are fully developed and the baby's visual perception is underdeveloped. Although growth takes place rapidly, the adult state of un-fuzzy vision is not reached until a child is five years old. The eye muscles and the system of linkage which coordinates movements of both eyes together are not fully developed until a child is eight.

Poor eyesight

The human lens has only a limited capacity to alter its focal length. If the eyeball is either too long or too short the image will not fall sharply on to the retina. This happens with long sight, when the eyeball is too short, and with short sight, when the eyeball is too long. Clouding of the lens, or cataract, will blur the image. A deformity of the window of the eye, the cornea, will distort the image – this is known as astigmatism and is sometimes found to go hand-in-hand with short sight.

41

Not being able to see very well does not have a great effect on a child's capability of learning to read. Of course, severe partial sighted-ness or total blindness are major handicaps, but the schoolchild with astigmatism or short sight does remarkably well. Parents should re-member that a lot of defects of vision may not be obvious at the age of five when the child first goes to school, but may develop later. Make sure that your child does have his regular eye examinations. If he has missed them for some reason, for instance because he has had mumps or flu, his eyes should be checked when he is better.

The real handicap for the child with uncorrected poor vision comes when he cannot see the blackboard or the cricket ball well. It is easy to assume that because your child passed his first eye test satisfactor-ily, there is nothing wrong with his eyesight. If later, at the age of eight or over, he is doing badly at school, another cause may be found and assumed to be the sole reason for his problems. This is the time to recheck his eyesight. There is no sense in a child being short-sighted and dyslexic, and not getting at least the short sight corrected.

You and his teacher will need to persuade your child to wear his glasses. Adults forget how uncomfortable their first pair of spectacles felt. Teasing in the playground is inevitable – 'Four eyes, four eyes, four eyes!' Your child will need a lot of support, encouragement and dis-cipline if he is going to go on wearing his glasses, and therefore be able to see well.

Colour vision defects, which are commoner in boys than girls, are not usually regarded as being much of a handicap when it comes to learning to read and spell, though colour blindness may be of import-ance if the teacher decides to use an elaborate colour-coded teaching system. Poor colour vision may be of great importance when it comes to deciding on a career. All sorts of jobs require high standards of colour vision. So before you encourage your child in his chosen ambition, make sure that his colour vision is of an acceptable standard. Sensitivity to colours or bright light may be a contributory cause of dyslexia.

To sum up: if glasses are prescribed for your child, make sure he wears them; if he has poor colour vision, make sure the teacher knows. By far and away the commonest form of visual impairment amongst schoolchildren is short sight for which glasses have been prescribed but are not worn.

Jennifer was one of identical twins born five weeks early. She had been an easy baby, had walked at nine months and talked sentences around her third birthday. A speech therapist consulted at the time did not suggest any treatment. Her successive schools remained unworried, but when she got to her comprehensive school her mother noticed that, unlike her twin, she could neither spell nor tackle unfamiliar words. Aged twelve when she came to the clinic, Jennifer had the reputation of being 'very physical' (she was a good swimmer), and of not taking life seriously. Her mother assured us that her school reports were good. She was a little shy, cheerful and went through all the tests vigorously. Her literacy attainments were a full three years below what was expected at her age and her oral receptive language weaker still. She turned out to be very short-sighted, especially in the left eye, but she admitted cheerfully that she never wore her glasses. Her visual sequential memory [102] was poor, her expressive language scant, she had slight trouble with articulation and a poor auditory sequential memory [73]. However, her IQ was in the average range [67]. The speech therapist offered a programme to help with auditory sequential memory, the teacher suggested language activities and gave her a reading list. Everyone agreed that she ought to wear her glasses all the time. Six weeks later she was still not wearing them. Could her teachers be asked to remind her at the start of every lesson, even if she didn't want to wear them in the street? Oh no, said her mother, her school must not know that an outside opinion had been sought.

Squinting

A squint is a failure of binocular vision. The eyes do not fix on the same target and may point inwards or outwards. There are many different causes, some of them associated with poor reading. Illnesses affecting the brain, diseases of the eye muscles or nerves controlling them, inflammation and subsequent bandaging of one eye are examples of possible causes of squint. The exact coordination of the eyes needed to develop binocular vision may never be achieved by a child with severe difficulty in learning; it is not surprising that a higher proportion of squints is found among children of very low intelligence than in the general population.

42

Some children have times when they squint, and if this is allowed to go on unchecked it may eventually turn into a permanent deviation of one eye. Watch out for the child who always squints when he becomes very excited – he tends to squint inwards, as compared with the lethargic child who may squint outwards. A useful clue that a child may be developing a squint is frequent or persistent head-tilting. If this starts happening or you can see a squint, consult your doctor. The eye specialist and the orthoptist together will treat the squint and will get better results the earlier they see the child. If allowed to squint unchecked, the child will use only his good eye and suppress what he sees with the squinting eye. Eventually he will lose all vision in the bad eye. This is a danger which threatens the squinting child until he is about seven.

Wobbly eyes

There is a condition which can prevent a squinting child from developing normal binocular vision even after treatment. Our eyes wobble if we look out of a train window as the telegraph poles flash by. This is quite normal. Some people are born with a persistent eye-wobble; *nystagmus* is the technical word for it. It may also happen as the result of some disease process. To the onlooker, the child's eyes flicker slightly all the time. They may fix for the moment on some target and then they are off again, trembling like a dog's nose scenting something delicious.

43

Nystagmus by itself is not a cause of dyslexia, though some of the underlying diseases may be. If it is associated with poor vision, it may make things extra difficult in the classroom.

Peter was a delightful character, bright, chatty and friendly. He had had a stormy birth; the cord had been round his neck and he was a bit blue on arrival. Initially he was a quiet baby, rather slow to feed. From the early days it was obvious that he had a squint and congenital nystagmus – he was born with wobbly eyes. The squint was corrected by an operation.

When he went to school he did quite well at first, but then when he was nearly seven he got a new form teacher. His progress suddenly began to drop off.

He was referred to the clinic for assessment, but his mother solved the problem for him just before he came. She recognized that in order to see more clearly, he always reduced eye-wobble by looking hard to the right, thus fixing his eyeballs at least temporarily. To do this in class, he was used to sitting on the left of the class and turning his head and trunk to the left, so looking out of the corner of his eye. The new teacher had put him on the right of the class. Result – disaster. Repositioning cured his problem.

Patterns of print

44 New research work suggests that three eye problems, which may reflect some slight degree of abnormal brain function, are relevant to dyslexia. Firstly, for some adults, several lines of print on a page form a pattern which gives eye-strain, headaches and even illusions of colour, shape and movement. The underlying mechanism seems to be akin to that which produces epileptic-type attacks in some of us if we look at a persistently flickering TV screen [120]. Adults who get such attacks benefit from using a shield to block out all the lines of print on a page except the one they are reading. It is tempting to think that some children may also be suffering from eye-strain and headaches from looking at patterns of print. However, the research work to confirm this has not yet been done, and until it has, it is wrong to jump to any conclusions.

Secondly, glare can make reading uncomfortable. Glare is the oppressive shine coming off a page which is brightly lit in contrast to the room around it. It is the contrast in illuminations between the target and the surroundings which results in glare. Too much glare can produce eye-strain, headaches and a reluctance to look at the page for very long. Levelling-out the contrast between the light on the page and the light in the room relieves the glare. Relief comes either by making the room brighter, or more commonly, by dimming the brightness of the page. This can be achieved by covering the page with a sheet of transparent coloured material or the eyes with tinted glasses. The extent to which this problem may affect school children has yet to be investigated fully, and much more research work needs to be done to evaluate this problem, and its relation to the one above.

Thirdly, there are children who get muddled when scanning print, jumping from one line to another and getting the order in which they read letters wrong. This is normal up to the age of eight and a finger under the target word is the usual aid to accurate reading. However, if these problems persist, the child should see an eye specialist, that is an oculist or an ophthalmic surgeon, for possible referral to an orthoptist. Part of the routine screening of children who are slow to read should be that they see an orthoptist. She will check vision and make sure that both eyes are working together satisfactorily. If she finds something wrong, she may give the child exercises or may prescribe glasses with one lens frosted and the other clear, to be worn only when the child is reading. In such an event she will tell you that the child's 'reference eye' is not well established yet. Most of us have learnt to pay attention to the signals received from one eye only when we read. Children should have developed this habit by the age of eight. Often the reference eye is established in a few months and the child can then abandon the use of the glasses. If such treatment is prescribed, be sure to attend the orthoptist when she asks to see your child again. Do not let the treatment run on unsupervised. Unhappily in our experience, the establishment of the reference eye is only very rarely associated with an improvement in reading. A case history will serve to draw the general picture.

Matthew was in a terrible state of nerves. At the age of ten, he was conscious that he was bad at reading. Everyone else agreed with him. His I Q had been estimated; he was of bright average intelligence. He was given remedial help at school; it did not help. His parents paid for extra teaching during the holidays; that did not help either. His vision had been tested at the routine school medical examination; it was all right. But Matthew complained of headaches, blurred vision and stomach-aches, and of seeing double. A diagnosis of migraine was made and he was not allowed chocolate. His condition got worse. Finally he said he could not see at all. The ophthalmologist found nothing wrong with his eyes and referred him to the orthoptist. He did not have an established reference eye. Interestingly enough, he seemed to attempt some sort of self-treatment. When reading, he put his head on his left arm, thus using one eye only. This had produced the usual adult reaction: 'Sit *up* when you read.' The orthoptist gave him the appropriately blanked-out glasses. Three months later, his reference eye was established, his headaches and double vision had gone and his reading was improving. The school reported that he was a different boy.

A warning: Not all cases are quite so easy and an unestablished reference eye is not a common cause of learning disability.

Summary (38–44)

Normal vision contributes to the child's experience of the world around him.

Poor eyesight has little impact on a child's ability to learn to read.

Poor eyesight does affect a child's performance in the classroom because he may not be able to see the blackboard.

In spite of normal eyesight, faulty illumination of a page, causing glare, may make it difficult for a child to read for long.

By eight a child should be using one eye only to read with. This is his reference eye. Failure to establish a reference eye may have some bearing on a few children's ability to learn to read.

An orthoptist will correct an unestablished reference eye, but this does not always correct the reading problem.

If glasses are prescribed for your child, you must make sure that he uses them.

Above all, if you think that there is something wrong with your child's eyes, see a doctor before embarking on any vision or eye movement training.

Chapter Five
Other Sensations

Introduction

Vision and hearing are not the only sensations which we may experience. Touch, temperature, pain, limb position, movement and the pull of gravity are all recorded; information from the special sense organs is relayed to the central nervous system. Such a mass of stimuli arriving all at once must be sorted and made meaningful. Not everything reaches consciousness, but what does must still be divided into important matter to be used and unimportant matter which can be ignored.

Experience derived from all these sensations plays a major role in our daily perception of the world around us and of our own physical position in it at any one time.

The tiny child is protected from this overwhelming bombardment of incoming stimuli by the underdevelopment of his brain cell systems [62, 63]. Increasing neurological maturity enables him to learn and to develop, but by the same token he cannot do more than his level of growth, his age, will permit. It is no good trying to push your child's development along faster than is normal. It is fine to develop his capabilities, but a mistake to try to get him to do what those capabilities will not permit.

Movement, gravity and balance

Almost part of the inner ear, but having nothing to do with hearing, are the semicircular canals (see Figure 1), three looped tubes set at right angles to one another and situated near the 'spiral staircase' [25]. Each canal contains fluid and a sensor at one end. The whole complex is known as the vestibular system.

Changes in direction (or in the speed of movement) of the head set up currents in the fluid and these stimulate the sensor. Nerve fibres carry the information from these sensors to the mid-brain [58]. From there it travels either up to the cerebellum [59] and the cerebral cortex [54], or downwards to the spinal cord and to the limbs.

The information received enables us to recognize when we are

45

moving, changing direction or stopping. Not all of it reaches consciousness. Some of it is relayed to the centres controlling the rest of the body. The stimuli are integrated with messages coming in from the eyes, ears and receptors of sense of position of the limbs to enable balance and direction of movements to be maintained.

At one time it was firmly believed that there was a direct relationship between an innate weakness of this integratory system and dyslexia. Accepting this concept, it was logical to attempt to improve integration and therefore the ability to read by physical stimulation. Programmes using stimulation of touch by stroking, or stimulation of the vestibular system by spinning, were devised. As well as improving a child's general awareness it was hoped that there would be a direct impact on the reading abilities of the learning-disabled child. Subsequent studies have not really substantiated the underlying belief of the direct connection between poor sensory integration and dyslexia [131].

This does not mean that such programmes are useless. There is often a collateral, rather than a causative, problem which is relieved, and there is no doubt that all children, whether they be learning-disabled or not, benefit from, enjoy and are stimulated by the activities.

Programmes designed to stimulate sensory integration, body awareness, sense of position and competent movement should be seen as promoting general awareness and not as cures for dyslexia. The case of Walter serves to illustrate the benefit and the misconceptions which may result when a child is helped by a course of physical therapy.

Walter came to the clinic when he was seven years and ten months because he was at least one year behind his peers in everything at school, despite special teaching four times a week. In her report his remedial teacher noted that he often 'drifted away', so that questions and instructions had to be repeated, that he had difficulty telling sounds apart, more difficulty with the shapes and orientation of letters and absolutely no idea of number. His medical history disclosed a threatened abortion at about the ninth week of pregnancy, which kept his mother in bed for the next six weeks, followed by premature birth after prolonged labour. He had been a very noisy baby, who resisted solid food and had frequent bouts of high temperature.

Formal testing revealed trouble on all fronts: balance, coordination, ability to follow instructions for movement, orientation in space and sense of rhythm were exceptionally poor. He mispronounced words, took a long time to understand and answer questions, and his auditory sequential memory [73] was at rock bottom. His visual sequential memory and discrimination were little better; his handwriting, with a tightly clenched and inadequately controlled pencil, was dreadful: letters were often rotated right to left, whether he was copying or writing to dictation one letter at a time or whole words. He could sound out ('bark at') print up to a point but he didn't understand what he read. His parents said he had always been very clumsy. But his vision and hearing were up to scratch and his I Q average [67].

A joint operation was decided upon: the physiotherapist saw him once a week for exercises. These she accompanied by a rhyming libretto, so that her words related to his actions, helping him to monitor the movements. The rhythm of her commentary and the predictability of the rhymes were intended also to start work on his poor auditory memory, an extra to the obvious aim of encouraging kinetic melody as distinct from his habitual jerky movements. The speech therapist, in consultation with the occupational therapist, advised the parents what games to play with him at home; the teacher recommended cursive writing and several types of comprehension games and exercises, mostly oral.

Four months later improvement was apparent: balance and coordination were so greatly improved that the school's normal physical education programme could be left to take over their development; his pencil-hold was normal, his handwriting cursive [192], letter rotations had dropped by three-quarters and spelling improved dramatically; understanding of what he read had soared well ahead of his chronological age. The speech therapist decided to give him a short intensive course to improve his organization of auditory–verbal material; the occupational therapist found his visual sequential memory had greatly improved and she suggested more games to be played at home. His mother remarked on how much less clumsy he was.

A year later Walter passed an exam for entry into an academic school attended by his elder brothers. Six years later he had done the first batch of public exams (O-levels) with success and was a confident, cheerful lad who had just discovered the joys of wind-surfing. His mother was still convinced that the initial exercises for balance and coordination had been the key to all the other advances – which was undervaluing the roles played by the speech therapist and remedial teacher, but what matter from Walter's point of view?

Skin

46 If the eyes and ears are the early-warning units of the body's defences, the skin is the network of outposts in front of the main line.

The skin contains a myriad of sense organs which record pain, touch and changes in temperature and pressure. They are to be found in the greatest numbers where they are most needed. The highest concentrations are in the lips and fingers. It is easier to tell how far apart two sharp points (perhaps on a compass) may be by using your fingertip rather than your shoulder. If you want to know more about an unfamiliar object, you finger it rather than sit on it.

In addition the skin plays a part in temperature control, the blood vessels beneath it acting like a radiator in hot weather or constricting to cut down the flow of hot blood and thus conserving heat on cold days. Inadvertently they may play a part in body language, producing the pallor of fear or flushing the skin by dilating with embarrassment.

Perhaps none of this has much to do with learning disabilities, though there are one or two diseases to consider.

Eczema, EFAs and zinc

47 Eczema is a red, intensely irritating rash which mainly affects the inside surfaces of the skin over the elbows or knees, the hands and the face. Patches of eczema may be raw and weeping or thickened and cracked. The intense itching can make a child 'tear himself to pieces'. When under emotional pressure, the child with eczema scratches incessantly.

Eczema is a common manifestation of allergy (sometimes called atopy), hay fever, asthma and some forms of migraine and nettle rash being others.

There is some evidence that hyperactivity [134] and eczema go together, and that in some such cases improvement may result if the child is given 'essential fatty acids' or 'EFAs'.

Essential fatty acids are a form of fat which the body needs but cannot make for itself, in contrast with ordinary fat which is made out of carbohydrates (sugar and flour) if we eat too much. These EFAs are found in several vegetable oils, one of the richest sources being evening primrose oil. To make effective use of them, the body has to change them once they are absorbed and the chemical processes involve the use of zinc.

Zinc, too, is essential to the body's chemistry. It is present in the normal diet, mainly in animal constituents rather than in vegetables. Inadequate levels of zinc in the body may result from various conditions: there may be a congenital inability to use it; there may be not enough in a vegetarian diet; there may be faulty absorption from the gut; there may be increased loss due to bowel disease.

An acute shortage of zinc produces a florid red rash, which is usually symmetrical, on the face, head, buttocks, arms, elbows and knees – but it isn't eczema. The patients may go bald, have eye irritation and be weak and lethargic.

Of much more interest is the mild, sub-acute form of zinc deficiency, in which there may be behaviour problems, a low growth rate and less than normal amounts of zinc in the blood and hair.

Just how important the interplay of EFAs, zinc, eczema and hyperactivity is in the production of learning disabilities is not certain. Before jumping to the conclusion that all a child's schoolroom problems can be solved by feeding him the oil of the evening primrose, it is important to check for all the other possible causes of learning disabilities and disorders. So do not put your child on to any sort of unusual diet unless his paediatrician recommends that you should. Never 'go it alone'; always get medical advice first.

Threadworms

Threadworms live in the human rectum, just inside the anus, and come out at night to lay their eggs round the back passage. If the eggs are carried to the mouth, either via fingers scratching the back passage or from a carpet or bedding on to which they have fallen, then they hatch inside and another generation of worms begins. They tickle. This keeps a child awake at night and may make him wriggle around in class, easing the irritation by rubbing his bottom on the chair seat. He is listless because of the lack of sleep and inattentive because of the tickle. Occasionally, the label of hyperactivity [134] is attached to him, followed by the query, 'Could he be dyslexic?' A rash is visible around the anus and swabbing with a piece of sticky cellophane picks up the eggs which can be identified in a laboratory. The cure for threadworms must be taken by the whole family for, as like as not, someone else has them as well; if they are not eradicated from all possible reservoirs, they return as the eggs are picked up after treatment is finished. Finger-

48

sucking and mouthing toys do not help, because eggs can be carried in these ways, but no one ever managed to stop their child putting his fingers in his mouth and it is better to attack the worms than the child.

All children suspected of having learning disabilities or learning disorders should be undressed, otherwise something medically important will be missed. The possibility of threadworms is a good example of the need for a doctor to examine the child thoroughly.

Helen was one of the best-turned-out little girls we had ever seen. She arrived with both parents and a tentative diagnosis of hyperactivity, made by her mother. She was doing badly at school; when she had started at five all had gone well, but now that she was eight she was getting bad reports. She was irritable, a cross-patch, did not pay attention in class ('Helen must try to concentrate') and was drowsy towards the end of the day. Her mother said she slept badly – always thrashing about in her bed – 'We can hear her on the go when we go up to bed ourselves.' 'When did she last see your doctor?' (a routine question). 'Well, she has this rash down below and she has some cream for that.' A quick look at her back passage revealed the presence of an obliging worm which appeared at just the right moment.

Then followed the difficulty of persuading the family that, firstly, threadworms were irritating things which make any child overactive and, secondly, that they were a family disease as well as a child's one. Her father was warned that the stem of his pipe was an effective vehicle for threadworm eggs, which could hitch a lift on it from some infested area via his mouth to their incubation site in his intestine.

Treatment was started for the whole family, father included. He switched to cigarettes and was almost persuaded to give up smoking when it was pointed out that his fingers could also be egg transporters.

Asthma

49 The asthmatic child has bouts of wheezing when he cannot breathe out properly and may be very distressed indeed. The attacks may come suddenly. The cause may be an allergic response to something specific like cat dandruff or some pollens. Frequently the attacks are fired off by infections and are easily started by colds. Brisk exercise makes some children wheeze. Bad attacks are very frightening for both the child and his parents. It is common practice to keep the child from school either to allow him to recover from an attack or for fear that, if there are a lot of colds about, he might get one.

There is no evidence that asthma is directly associated with learning disabilities. However, the repeated brief absences from school which a child with persistent asthma suffers do have a marked effect on his learning. Precise inquiry about the number of days he has missed from school because of his asthma may reveal that an asthmatic child has been away for twenty-five per cent of the school year – enough to damage his chances of keeping up with the other children and enough to justify extra help to enable him to catch up. The parents should seek advice from their doctor about the treatment of minor attacks and about the value of keeping him off school.

Chapter Six
The Brain

Introduction

It is easy to think of the brain as a super-computer put together by cherubim in some celestial silicon-chip valley. This would be a mistake because printed circuits, however microscopic, are not alive and the brain is.

In spite of the multitude of books and papers written about it, we are still remarkably ignorant of the brain's functions. We do better when it comes to its anatomy because generations of doctors who knew too much Greek or Latin and not enough physics or chemistry spent a lot of time giving all the parts difficult names. Reference has to be made to this geography of the brain so that local diseases or local functions can be put into some sort of perspective. This section will deal with the anatomy and structure of the brain and touch briefly on function, to set the scene for the one that follows on brain damage. (See Chapter 10.)

The anatomy of the brain

50 There are three main parts to consider: the cerebrum; the mid-brain; and the cerebellum. Figure 3 shows, in the form of a diagram, a head cut in half from top to bottom. In it you can see the cerebrum on top, the mid-brain which looks like a stalk and the cerebellum tucked under the back part of the cerebrum behind the mid-brain.

The cerebrum

Chip off the vault of the skull as you would chip off the top of your breakfast egg and you will see the cerebrum exposed. It looks like a large walnut and, like a walnut, is divisible into two symmetrical halves, called the right and left cerebral hemispheres. Inside each hemisphere are interconnecting spaces, the ventricles, filled with cerebrospinal fluid. The surface of the cerebrum is called the cortex. It is marked by fissures and cracks which give it its walnut-like appearance and also serve as the boundary lines of the subdivisions or lobes. There are four principal lobes in each hemisphere – frontal, parietal, temporal and

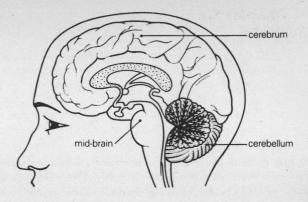

Figure 3   A section through the head

occipital (see Figure 4). In general, the right cerebral hemisphere deals with the left half of the body and the left cerebral hemisphere with the right half. Leashes of nerve fibres – rather like telephone cables – run down from the cerebral cortex. They pass either just to the opposite hemisphere, or, on more of a downward run, to the mid-brain and cerebellum and eventually to the spinal cord.

The mid-brain

The mid-brain is an inverted cone or solid cornet on which the cerebrum sits, like a double ice-cream. It runs downwards to become the spinal cord, and carries the fibres from the cerebrum to other parts of the body and the fibres from other parts of the body to the cerebrum. It has nerve centres of its own, each with its own function. Most of the nerves supplying the muscles of the head and carrying information from the main sense organs in the head run out of or into the mid-brain.

The cerebellum

The cerebellum is about the size of a child's fist and is shaped like a Spanish chestnut. Its surface is heavily pleated, as are the tight petals of an old-fashioned rose. It receives bundles of nerve fibres both from the cerebral hemispheres and from the centres in the mid-brain related to hearing and vision. In its turn, the cerebellum sends fibres to muscle control centres, to the mid-brain and the cerebrum.

Summary (50)

There are three main parts of the brain: cerebrum, mid-brain and cerebellum (Figure 3).

The cerebrum is divided into left and right cerebral hemispheres.

Each hemisphere has four lobes: frontal, parietal, temporal and occipital (Figure 4).

The mid-brain sits below the hemispheres.

The cerebellum lies behind the mid-brain and under the cerebrum.

Brain tissues

51 The brain is made up of grey and white matter. The grey matter contains the large main cells, or neurons, and several different sorts of smaller cells, the glia or glue cells. There are about thirty billion main cells and approximately seven times as many glue cells. The white matter consists of fibres connecting one part of the brain with another, and of more fibres which run down the spinal cord. There is a network of blood vessels. The arteries bring oxygen, essential food supplies and sometimes unexpected chemicals to the brain cells. The artery network is like a tree whose branches get smaller and smaller, finally ending up as twigs, as they approach the particular area they supply with blood. The majority of these very fine blood vessels are the only means of bringing oxygen to a specific piece of brain tissue.

Brain cells

Neurons

52 Each neuron has: a cell body; a long fibre, the axon, down which the impulses travel away from the cell body; and a variable number of branching fingers, dendrites, which accept incoming impulses from other cells. (See Figure 5.)

Each axon is usually coated in an insulating sheath which increases the speed with which an impulse may travel down it. This coat is made from a waxy white substance, myelin, which gives the white matter its characteristic appearance. The axon ends in a bulb containing a lot of minute bubbles full of a chemical. Between the axon bulb and the next cell is a space. This system is called the synapse (see Figure 6). The chemical from the bubbles can travel across the synapse space, when it has been released by an electrical discharge coming down the axon. The chemical then excites the receptor plate of the next cell and starts a message travelling up its dendrite. It is then re-absorbed into the bubbles and there is a special blocking mechanism to stop it stimulat-

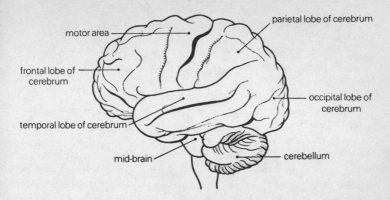

Figure 4   The left side of the brain

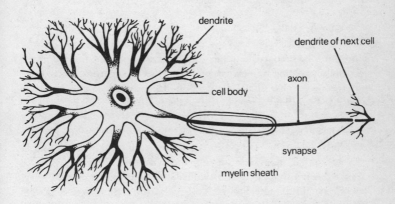

Figure 5   A brain cell – the neuron

ing its own parent cell. So the message starts in the body of one neuron, flows down its axon, crosses the synaptial space, on to the receptor plate of the next cell's dendrite and up into the cell's body, where it

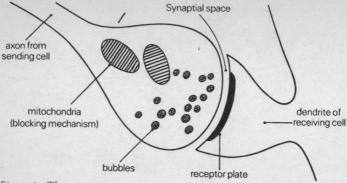

Figure 6   *The synapse*

may be boosted on its way to another cell in the chain (see Figure 7). There are several different chemical systems controlling the passage of messages from one cell to the next, some stimulating and others inhibiting the receptor cell. Drugs prescribed by doctors work at the synapse on these chemical systems and produce a desired effect by interference with one or more stages of the process.

Glue or glial cells
The glue or glial cells have several functions. Some lay down the sheaths of myelin which coat the axons and help to maintain them. Others form the supporting framework which carries the neurons. In contrast with these neurons, glial cells can divide and replace themselves if damaged. They play no part in the passage of messages.

The neuron chain
The cell body – axon – synapse – dendrite – cell body link can and is repeated, so that an impulse starting in one cell body may travel a long distance down a chain made of similar links. Many neurons have more than one synaptic connection with neighbouring cells. In fact, a neuron may have as many as ten thousand such contacts. If you recall that there are about thirty billion neurons in a brain, this makes quite a lot of synapses. The neuron chain is more often part of a network rather than a simple line, especially in the cerebral cortex. Any particular cell may be a way-station on more than one chain, receiving or sending messages to and from other cells. Some of these messages may be in the nature of 'stop' commands, others may indicate 'go'. The axons bundle together to form tracts, or leashes, of nerve fibres which run from the

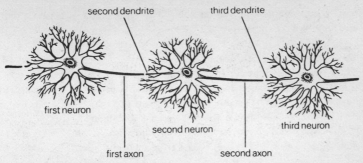

Figure 7   The neuron chain

higher brain centres to the various parts of the body which they supply with instructions. Similarly, information coming from the various sense organs (such as the touch buds; pain sensors; the receptors which record muscle movements, pressures on the body, heat, cold and vibrations – not to mention vision, hearing and smell) travels in bundles of nerve fibres up to the brain.

Summary (51–2)
The brain is made up of grey and white matter.
The grey matter contains thirty billion main cells (neurons) and even more supporting cells (glia).
A neuron can send messages down its main fibre (axon) to other cells.
The connection between two cells is called the synapse.
Transmission of impulses from one cell to another is carried out by chemical systems.
Medicines can act at the synapse to affect brain function.

Brain function
Years of study have been devoted to the adult brain, particularly in the comparison of it with those of various animals and also in the observation of brain-damaged patients both in life and after death. Detailed maps have been drawn, showing this or that part of the adult brain to be responsible for this or that function. It is easy to attribute too much importance to these maps and to forget that each part of the brain has an effect on all the others. Identified areas and their functions must not be seen in isolation. In the context of learning disabilities, it must also be remembered that the developing brain of a child is quite different

53

from the developed brain of an adult. Too close parallels between the one and the other must not be drawn.

Functions of the cerebrum

54 The outer lining of the cerebral hemisphere is called the cerebral cortex. It is easy to get at, either by surgery or with simple electrical measuring devices which may be used in the Outpatients department of a hospital. As a result, much is known about the effects of damage to specific areas of the cortex and about the functions of those areas. The left cerebral hemisphere has different capabilities from the right.

The left cerebral hemisphere

55 The left cerebral hemisphere is involved with communication, both by voice and by hand signals. In it are those areas which deal with sensations from and instructions to the right side of the body. It has control over mouth and hand movements not concerned with communication; the areas responsible lie mainly in the frontal lobe.

An injury to the frontal lobe may result in weakness of the right side of the body and perhaps some impairment of speech – the greater the extent of the damage, the greater the loss of function. Hearing, receptive speech and verbal reasoning are located in the temporal lobe, while reading, writing and some of the mechanical aspects of arithmetic are sited in the parietal one. The occipital lobe deals with stimuli from the right halves of the fields of vision of both eyes, together with some analysis of the messages received visually and with information about eye movements.

It is recognized that a right-handed adult has a dominant left cerebral hemisphere; most of us are right-handed; only ten per cent consider ourselves to be left-handed. Though ninety per cent are right-handed, only two-thirds are both right-handed and right-eyed. This means that there are more left-eyed people than there are left-handed ones. Some of us have mixed hand/eye dominance but do not necessarily have a learning disability [3]. While on this subject, it is important to appreciate that there is a difference between the dominant eye and the reference eye. (This topic is explored in section 44.) Because dominance of the left cerebral hemisphere and the presence of language centres in it occur in right-handed people, it might seem logical to assume that the language centres of left-handed people are always sited in the right cerebral hemisphere. This is not always the case. Ninety-seven per cent of right-handed people have left cerebral hemisphere dominance and left-sided language centres. Only sixty per cent of left-handed people have their language centres in the right halves of their brains. To complicate matters, very early unilateral brain damage may cause a shift of dominance, and of the speech and language centres, from an originally dominant side to the other.

The right cerebral hemisphere

The right cerebral hemisphere contains those areas which deal with sensations from and instructions to the left side of the body. In general, its functions are related to the recognition of shapes, visual and visuo-spatial perception and the construction of shapes, as in drawing. There is some mystery about the role of the frontal lobe. Hearing and music are served by the temporal lobe and the perception and appreciation of space by the parietal one.

56

The occipital lobe deals with stimuli from the left halves of the fields of vision of both eyes, together with some analysis of the messages received visually and with information about eye movements.

Damage to the right hemisphere may disturb the recognition of objects, even though they can still be seen clearly, or may affect the ability to recognize something even though its component parts are identified.

There has been a suggestion that hormonic influences in foetal life may promote the dominance of the right cerebral hemisphere at the expense of the left.

Reading and the two cerebral hemispheres

When they first start to read, most children use the shape recognition strengths of the right hemisphere because they need to pay close attention to the visual features of unfamiliar print. They see words and groups of letters as patterns, which give direct access to meaning. Meaning/semantics being part of language, the language skills of the left hemisphere act like a safety net into which these visual patterns fall. Children read accurately and slowly at this stage; their slowness is accepted and causes no comment.

57

This first visual approach accounts for most early reading schemes being 'look-and-say' (even if the words are phonically controlled, they are also chosen for their distinctive visual pattern). They are highly repetitive too. This gives frequent exposure to a limited number of patterns/words in a series of shifting contexts.

But at the same time as they start to read, children start to write. Initially the two activities are separate. To amalgamate them, the child is asked to read back what he has written on a topic of his choice. He still uses his visual strengths to retrieve the spoken form of the written pattern, but he is helped by the words of the pattern being important to him personally. Because he is writing, he is being taught patterns of hand movement needed for the formation of letters. While the former are much less important than visual patterns, they tend to underline the regularity of patterns and therefore their predictability.

When form and shape are mastered – that is, when a goodly number of words/patterns are recognized without conscious effort, the linguistic skills of the left hemisphere are brought into greater use. Meaning has underpinned the enterprise from the start and is now used to process larger visual patterns more quickly. Phonological analysis – analysing words for their patterns of sound–symbol association – also comes into its own. This is used for reading unfamiliar words and is also applied closely to spelling. Some phonic reading schemes are used, and reading generally speeds up and becomes less accurate.

Older children and adults use phonological analysis and organization for reading when the visual pattern of the word is not recognized and its meaning not evident from the context. Overall, experienced readers use both visual and linguistic strategies when reading. Visual memory predominantly controls spelling, helped out by the mastery of handwriting recurring letter combinations, which in their turn contain phonological and grammatical patterns.

So, since we read with both hemispheres – starting predominantly with the right, going on to predominantly the left, and spell predominantly with the right throughout – a nice balance between the two is vital. If the balance is tilted towards one or the other, one or other set of strategies is mainly used, to the greater or lesser detriment of reading progress.

Functions of the mid-brain

58 The mid-brain is the control centre for various automatic functions which operate from the word go: it ensures that the heart beats as it should, that food passes through the gut without too much fuss, that breathing happens sufficiently often for the needs of the moment. The mid-brain exercises control over three other important functions. The first is the wakefulness or sleepiness of the cerebral cortex. It ensures that incoming stimuli do not run riot over the cerebral hemispheres, but are dealt with in an orderly fashion. The second function is reminiscent of that of a 'spaghetti junction' on a motorway: where the nerve fibres from the cerebral hemispheres cross over, they must reach their destinations in spite of having started on the opposite side of the body. The third function is that of coordination, control of which is split between

74

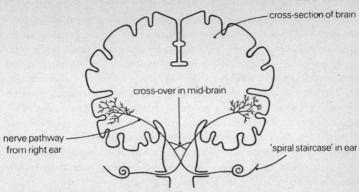

Figure 8   Nerve pathways from ear to brain

the mid-brain and the cerebellum. It seems to work out like this: between the conscious intention to do something like picking a pin off the floor and the achievement of that aim, there has to be selection of the muscles to be used, timing of their contractions and relaxations, and control of the amount of force expended. The mid-brain is concerned with the planning of the sequence of actions in the context of the need for a particular effect.

Functions of the cerebellum

The second coordinating system, located in the cerebellum, may remind readers familiar with LOGO of the simplest of its commands, that which brings user-defined procedure into action; for this second coordinating system seems to initiate already learnt programmes of coordinated action, particularly those concerned with hand skills. Further, and most importantly, it provides the necessary control of the rest of the body which enables the learnt programme to take place. You do not fall flat on your face when you bend forward to pick up that pin, because the cerebellum sees to it that you are properly balanced first. The cerebellum seems to create the stable muscle base from which more intricate movements take place. It is the coordinator of coordination.

59

Cross-overs

It is a peculiarity of the brain that each cerebral hemisphere gets its information from the opposite side of the body. Nerve pathways bringing impulses from the ears, eyes and limbs cross over in the mid-brain

60

before they end up in the cerebral cortex. The same thing happens to the bulk of fibres coming from that part of the cerebral cortex which gives instructions to the limbs. These cross-overs are not total.

Each ear sends impulses from the receptor cells of the 'spiral staircase' (the cochlea – see section 25) to the other side of the brain, but there is also some input to the same side via a smaller leash of nerve fibres. It is thought that, when sounds come into both ears simultaneously, the components which cross over to the other side of the brain suppress signals coming from the same side: a stereophonic system which results in the left cerebral cortex receiving, or rather hearing, signals from the right ear and vice versa for the right cerebral cortex (see Figure 8).

The visual pathways are somewhat similar. Everything seen in the left half of the left eye's field of vision, together with everything seen in the left half of the right eye's field of vision, end up being recorded by the right cerebral cortex. So the pathways from each retina only partially cross.

Sensations from, and instructions to, the hands and feet are almost completely crossed. What comes or goes from the right side of the brain starts or ends at the left side of the body – and, of course, the other way round for the left side of the brain. Do not forget these anatomical crossovers, otherwise you may get muddled when thinking about 'crossed laterals' [79].

Coordinated functions, or how things get done

61 Separating out each bit of the brain and itemizing its functions is an artificial process, but because of the brain's complexity some dissection is necessary for the sake of clarity. The mechanics of action can be separated from the more intellectual functions.

Unfortunately the medical profession has a confusing habit of taking a perfectly ordinary word, rejecting the meaning which we all understand (anyway on one side of the Atlantic), and imposing an accurate but more obscure meaning. Take the word 'motor'; to most of us in Great Britain this means a car, an automobile, or something to do with a car. To the doctors, it means anything to do with movement. To them, 'motor development' does not mean the change from the Model T to the V8. Not a bit of it. It is medical jargon for a child's increasing ability to do things.

The fully developed motor system, by means of which we can do those things we want to, is complex and involves many parts of the brain. Have you ever wondered how it is that, when you take the dog for a walk, the process of putting one foot in front of the other just happens? Conscious effort on your part is confined to the decision to do something; the actions which follow barely need thinking about.

It is probable that, when we have decided to do something, the brain selects a suitable programme which gives orders to the relevant muscles. These programmes have been born in us or have been learnt as we have been growing up. It is akin to a 'mystery' coach tour. Having decided to go, we get into the coach and the tour operator puts into action his pre-planned holiday programme. The programmes embedded in the nervous system are very specific. 'Walk' implies one programme, 'jump' another, 'stop' a third. Each fires off a whole sequence of muscle movements both to change the position of the limbs and to support those changes. Before the target movement is achieved, various levels of brain function must come into action. Each is located in a different part of the brain. The final movement may be affected in different ways if the component parts of the brain involved are diseased or damaged. At this point, have a look at Figure 4 (p. 69), which shows the names of the different brain parts, once again. It will refresh your memory.

The actual instructions to the limbs and muscles come from the motor area of the cerebral cortex, though the cerebellum provides important feedback information as movement is taking place. This feedback allows small local adjustments of posture to be made to fit in with local circumstances at the time. The cerebellum also plays a part in setting up the particular programme to be used, once it has been selected. It controls the selection of muscle groups, together with timing and the amount of force to be used. Part of the mid-brain is involved in the actual selection of the right programme necessary to achieve the desired goal. The frontal lobes define that goal and indicate what sort of programme will be necessary to get there. The parietal lobes provide information coming in from the different sense organs. This tells us what is happening outside the body, in particular about the space around us. It contributes to the functioning of the frontal lobes by indicating what should and can be done.

Finally, parts of the mid-brain and the inner cortical system make ready the voluntary action, start it off and keep a check to find out what is happening as it happens.

Summary (53–61)
Each cerebral hemisphere receives messages from, and gives instructions to, the opposite side of the body.
Together, the hemispheres deal with reading.

The right hemisphere deals with the shape of words.
The left hemisphere deals with their sounds.
A good balance between the two is essential for learning to
read.
The mid-brain controls the automatic functions of the body which
go on without our being aware of them: it controls the wakefulness of
the cerebrum; it coordinates body movements.
The cerebellum also coordinates body movements.

Development of the brain

62 Before birth there is a period of rapid cell multiplication, so that all the neurons are formed by the sixth month of foetal life. The future growth in size of the human brain does not mean an increase in the number of these cells. At and around the time of birth, there is a burst of cell growth when the glial cells increase in number. The brain gets bigger as myelin sheaths, which are few at birth, are laid down round the axons. This goes on steadily for the first two years of life. At the same time, there is an increase in the size of the neuron bodies and an increase in the number of dendrites. Therefore more synapses develop and greater intercommunication between cells is possible.

The source of energy for these bursts of growth comes from sugar and oxygen. When the child is in the womb, these are brought in the mother's blood and cross the placenta to reach the baby. After birth, he has to switch suddenly to absorbing sugar from his food and oxygen from the air he breathes. Without adequate supplies of food and oxygen, both in the womb, during birth and in the cot, his brain cells cannot develop, survive or grow. They are at their most vulnerable when they are growing most actively; that is when they need most nutriment. If they lack an adequate blood supply, or the blood supply is vitiated by poison in some form, trouble ensues. In the first instance, trouble consists of interference with the chemical processes by which the brain cells can use sugar and oxygen. In the second, brain cells can be killed or their growth prevented. In the final analysis, you see a child with a clearly defined disability.

Overall the developing brain of the child is not the same as the developed brain of the adult. The functions of the adult brain cannot develop in the child unless the brain systems have developed first. Reading must wait on cell system readiness. Energy starvation, from whatever cause, may hinder or prevent development of function.

Changes in brain function during development
The transition from infancy to adulthood has been studied by many distinguished authorities as well as by anxious parents. The Russian psychologist, Alexander Luria, and the Swiss psychologist, Jean Piaget, define developmental stages from different points of view which, when put together, give useful guidelines for parents and teachers concerned with learning difficulties.

63

Luria postulates that the brain has three functional systems: the first for regulating tone and waking the cerebral cortex; that is, of course, a mid-brain activity [58]. The second is for obtaining, processing and storing information; this is situated in the occipital, parietal and temporal lobes of both cerebral hemispheres. The third is for controlling mental activity, and is to be found in the frontal lobes.

Each of these three functional systems has within itself a similar structure of cell zones:

- a primary zone consisting of large neurons with long axons, each cell having very limited and specific functions;
- a secondary zone where the neurons are not so big and the axons not so long, but where there are more dendrites. Here, processing and preparing of programmes takes place;
- a tertiary zone in which all the neurons have short axons and where there is a great deal of intercommunication with other areas. Conscious activity is organized here.

In the adult brain, the tertiary zone is in control; we can select what we want to make use of from the multitude of incoming stimuli. While engaged in conversation with someone of interest to us, we hear and listen to what they have to say, discarding the noise of the passing aeroplane or car.

The situation is very different for the infant. Arriving suddenly in the world of noise and light, heat and cold, desperately in need of food to supply his relatively large brain with the wherewithal for growth and survival, the bombardment of stimuli would be overwhelming if he had a fully developed adult brain with all the myriad intercommunications between its cells. Fortunately, at birth the child's brain is not fully formed. All those dendrites which are so obvious in Luria's secondary zone have not yet developed; the myelin sheaths round the axons have not yet been made by the glia, so impulses do not travel as quickly as they will in adult life; the neurons have yet to grow bigger. So for a while the primary zone of Luria is dominant, supplying the secondary and tertiary zones with information to be stored as invaluable experience or useful programmes. The child sees everything but understands little. The adult may not understand much more, but he only sees what he wants to.

Piaget described three main stages of development. The first is that of sensorimotor development after birth, when one burst of brain growth is at its height, and the increase in dendrites and laying-down of myelin is taking place. During this time the baby switches from those primary reflex programmes so disliked by Dr Johnson ('Babies, Madam? I hate 'em, they do nothing but sneeze, fart and gurk') to become responsive, imitative and communicative. The primary zone of Luria is giving way to the tertiary one. This becomes even more evident when the child passes through what Piaget called 'the pre-operational stage' of building his own internal picture of the world outside. At the same time he cracks the language code of his mother tongue. This stage should be completed by the time he is seven. By the age of eleven, insulation of the long nerve fibres should be complete, the tertiary zone of Luria is firmly dominant and the youth can go into the overdrive of logical thinking.

All this may account for things in theory, but what parents need to know is what they should be seeing. Without knowing anything of the normal pattern of development, they cannot recognize delays or disorders for which they should seek advice. Chapter 7 outlines some aspects of the child's normal development which his parents should be able to witness.

Summary (62–3)
A baby's brain is smaller than an adult's.
A baby's brain needs lots of food and oxygen to grow.
Starvation or poisons can kill growing brain cells.
If too many cells are affected, obvious brain damage results.
Brain function depends on brain development.
If the cell systems are not ready, the baby's development cannot advance.
At first the infant sees, hears and feels everything, understands little and is busy learning and remembering.
Adults only hear and see what they want to, discarding unimportant information.
Adults remember the past and learn with an effort.
The infant has little past to remember and learns all the time.

Chapter Seven
Perception, Intelligence and Memory

Introduction

Between the visual, hearing and general sensory areas of the adult cerebral cortex lie the association areas. Information from the eyes and ears reaches the brain in simple form. Messages sent in from sensory organs are first received as lines of light or as isolated items of sound; these are identified by individual cells, each of which can perform only one function. Destroy one of the cells and the patient loses only a tiny component of a whole, not enough to alter his realization or perception of what he is looking at or listening to. The adult performs complex decoding of the incoming simple signals to extract information from them. Previous experience has taught him what they mean. As the impulses move across the cerebral hemispheres, the information from the initial receptor areas of the brain becomes woven into meaningful, recognizable patterns which reach consciousness. The exploitation of incoming basic information becomes increasingly complex as the message of sight, sound, touch, taste and balance are mixed together.

64

Damage, such as follows a stroke, to different parts of the adult brain produces different effects depending on the anatomical site affected. Some indication of the functions of an area can be obtained by studying the effects of the trauma. For example, near the reception centre for noises are three closely related zones. Damage to the first makes the patient deaf to the small units of sound which make up speech (phonemes) and there is weakening of his perception of speech sounds. He therefore has difficulty in interpreting speech. This is reflected in his reduced ability to name objects or to recall the right word for an object. He cannot write from dictation, but because the damage is all in the hearing part of the brain he can copy what he can see. There is no loss of the ability to cope with grammar (that is, the organization of words), visual perception and mathematics.

Damage to the second zone leaves the hearing of the individual phonemes intact, but the memory for even short series of sounds becomes poor. Long sentences are difficult to understand if they are spoken, but present little problem if written.

Damage to the third zone produces difficulty in naming objects and also in drawing them.

In another part of the brain – the parietal lobe [50] of the left cerebral hemisphere – damage may result in an inability to grasp the meaning of a sentence rather than the meaning of individual words. The component parts of something may be recognized, but cannot be perceived as a whole and so do not make sense. Take the capital letter A, for example: a patient as described above would know that there should be a horizontal line and two diagonals, but he will not be able to put them together. This defect extends to copying a letter while looking at it, as well as trying to write it from memory.

Damage as described in the two latter instances causes faulty perception, that is, faulty interpretation of stimuli. In turn this reduces the capability of expression.

The child, during his progress to maturity, has to pass from a state of initial ignorance to an adult state of knowledge. His perception must grow with every other faculty; the growth of perception is dependent on other systems (for example, the motor control of movement) developing at the same time; all the other systems contribute to the expansion and evolution of one another, as well as of perception. All these systems are not only mixed up with one another, but are also inter-related.

Parents need to know if the development of their child's perceptual ability is not progressing at a normal rate. It is particularly difficult to recognize this. Consider, for instance, the problem of measuring the spatial perception, which enables a child to match or differentiate between the shapes, sizes or positions of various shapes. This perception is the result of the processing of various inputs. It is easiest to find out what has gone in by observing what comes out, perhaps in the form of a drawing. But while trying to do that, the observer starts to test something else as well, namely constructional or visuo-motor capability. When a child is encouraged to put something on to paper, then not only are his perceptual processes tested but also his ability to reproduce what he has perceived. Not only the adult but the child as well may recognize that the latter's efforts are incorrect or imperfect. You may encourage him to try again and to do better. He may get upset because he can perceive that what he has produced is not the same as what he had hoped to draw (a feeling familiar to all would-be artists).

Parents need some indication of when they should seek help. In spite of the problems just mentioned, it is best for parents to look at what comes out – what their child can do – rather than to bother about what goes in and what happens inside. Paper, pencils, paint and puzzles form the background against which milestones can be registered.

If these milestones are not passed at about the right times, then seek help from the psychologists, together with the neurologists, and leave it to them to sort out the precise nature of your child's problem.

Developmental milestones of perception

65

Immediately after birth, a child has no grasp of the meaning of geometry. He has not had experience of the significance and language of forms, lines, angles and shapes in general. He cannot conjure up an image for himself and, even if he had the mechanical wherewithal, he cannot put that image on to paper. Development is dependent on a general exploration of space. The more effective this becomes, the more his drawings and brick-building activities improve. Not even the most optimistic parent will expect anything much in this field during the first twelve months of life.

But about the fifteenth month, if you arm your child with a paper and pencil and show him how to begin, he will scribble away. He will not produce anything meaningful to you, but he will attack the task almost with ferocity, perhaps with purpose and certainly with enthusiasm, although the result is not anything recognizable. He lacks both the visuo-spatial and motor development, together with the perceptual ability.

A few months later, he will be scribbing away all by himself and the scribbles will be becoming more circular.

By two and a half years, he can copy a T or a V, one way up or the other, and he will splash paint about in lines and dots. He is beginning to observe and the results show on paper, though he still has difficulty in making shapes.

The three-year-old can copy a circle and imitate a cross. He draws a man with a head and he can build a little bridge with three bricks. He can match yellow and red.

A four-year-old will build a small flight of steps with his bricks if you help him, and he can copy X, V, T, H and O. His picture of a man has a head, legs and trunk, with perhaps some features on the face. He will also draw a simple house if encouraged, but do not expect too much if you live in a big block of flats.

The five-year-old copies squares and triangles and may write some letters spontaneously. He may not worry too much about which way up the letters should be and he may be cavalier about crossing the

A. He can probably write his first name, if you have not saddled him with one containing too many letters. His man has a head, trunk, legs, arms and definitely some features on the face. His house has doors, windows, roof and chimney. He draws what he likes to draw over and over again. He should be able to match four colours and to name about ten. His perception of things is under way. He has entered the stage where the relationship of one thing to another matters – for example, there are usually two eyes to each head whether he has drawn it full face or in profile, so that it looks like something out of an Egyptian tomb. He puts into his drawing what he knows to be there, even if he cannot see it: 'That's the baby inside Mummy's tummy.' Knowledge of what is actually there overrides what can be seen from one viewpoint only. Do not be surprised if he draws all four sides of the house in the same plane so that you can see them all at once. Perspective, proportions and distance will not be reproduced on his paper until the age of nine – at that time he begins to draw a proper picture of what he sees. Less easy to pinpoint is a child's ability to distinguish figures from their background, to spot the camouflaged target. Fortunately, comics or the children's page of the dailies often contain puzzles in which you have to find the ice-cream cones hidden in the picture of a beach scene. 'How many fairy faces can you see among the trees?' 'See if you can spot Mickey Mouse's friends in this picture.' If your child is no good at doing this, it is not a reason for rushing off to see the doctor in a panic in case he is becoming dyslexic; but it can be a useful pointer, among others.

There is one time-honoured test which aims to measure the child's ability to spot the camouflaged target, the target being a simple geometric shape: a square, an oval, a kite shape, and so on. As the shapes become more difficult the distractors, the camouflage, become more obstructive. As in many other tests mentioned in this book, the child's ability is related to a developmental norm stretching up to the age of five or so. Hence a five-year-old may be said to perform like the average four-year-old. If an occupational therapist administers the test, her comments should be sought because from the teacher's point of view it is a fairly unsatisfactory investigation; it does not distinguish between the child's ability to hold in mind the shape he is seeking and his ability to match the held, imagined shape with comparable shapes among the distractors. The occupational therapist can shed light on the question of whether the child has forgotten what he is looking for, or whether he is unable to relate a square of given orientation and dimensions to squares of different sizes at different orientations. The relevance of this to reading is obvious: a child must be able to pick out a particular word or letter, regardless of its print size and its position on the page, in the line, in a bigger or longer word. There is the added complication of the reversible letters b, d, p, q and g; children face these only after the age of five, when of course they are taught to write them at the same time, so from the word go movement is brought in to aid this further level of perceptual development.

With older children, figure-ground difficulties can surface in relation to maps: the child cannot pick out from the welter of lines and signs on the page (or, worse still, the large sheet) the one he wants. But by the age of twelve or so he knows precisely where his trouble lies. In answer to a direct question he can tell whether he can, or cannot, remember the particular sign (for a church with a square tower, for instance), or whether, having remembered the sign, he is taking an inconveniently long time to locate it. Strategies for coping with either part of the problem are available.

In general, after the age of five – that is, once school has started – the child extends his ability to distinguish complex form and to take order and distance into account. Increasing experience of books and pictures enabled him to do this in 2D also. Experience of language helps him to exploit these through the imagination.

Poor visual perception can have a severe effect on a child's school performance.

Hugh was born all of a rush, his mother's labour being very short. He seemed well at first – a bit slow at sucking, perhaps, but otherwise well. However, it was soon obvious that he was clumsy; he had difficulty in feeding himself without making a mess. When he was given one of those toys in which different shapes can be posted into appropriate holes in a box, he could never get the right piece into the right slot. The idea that a round peg does not fit into a square hole never seemed to come his way. His parents tried hard to teach him and, in doing so, found that he did not know the difference between big and little and that he had no idea of size by the time he was four. He was always a sociable chap and he enjoyed his play-group a lot. School was a different matter. By the middle of the second term, he was always being kept back so that his teacher could give him some personal attention. He slept badly – his mother said she could hear him being angry in his sleep.

He was seen by the educational psychologist who found that he had an average I Q. This hid a discrepancy between his verbal I Q which was average, and his performance I Q which was low average. There was a 29-point difference [70]. Further psychological investigations confirmed that he had a marked weakness in visual perception. The psychologist referred him to the clinic for medical investigation.

When seen there at the age of seven years and two months, he seemed chatty but nervous, picking at himself and unable to sit still. The speech therapist found that his understanding of what was said to him was good, his auditory memory was normal and his discrimination of sounds satisfactory. He did have poor articulation, which she thought was probably indicative of a wider motor problem. The findings of the occupational therapist and the doctor confirmed this. Perhaps the most striking feature of his performance was his poor drawing of himself, which was just a heavy interlacing of curved pencil lines across the page – no form or figure was recognizable.

He was seen by the remedial teacher, the opening sentences of whose report read: 'This extremely likeable little boy was friendly, cooperative, articulate and beautifully mannered. His ambition is to be a footballer, a sensible choice in view of his inability to sit still.' His reading comprehension age [Neale, 165] was a year in advance of his chronological age, but his spelling was poor.

Medical investigations at this stage did not show anything significant that would enable the cause to be pinpointed.

However, things did not go smoothly. Over the years, his reading skills did not advance with age and his perceptual deficits became even more obvious. For example, when he was asked, at the age of eight and a half, to draw his family, he produced outline figures of his father, mother and two sisters, each with barely recognizable limbs and no features on the faces.

By the age of eleven, his incoordination had become very marked, and his electroencephalogram tracings [121], which had originally been normal, showed increasing generalized abnormalities. His reading was stuck at the eight-year-old level. He was still cheerful and outgoing, but prone to temper outbursts if put under educational stress – and who could blame him?

The local education authority had been closely involved at all stages and had offered maximum help, which had been supported by occupational therapy sessions in the holidays.

His case is typical of the ineffectiveness of everybody to help with visual perceptual problems. For younger children there are specific programmes, but for the older child there is not the same level of support as there is for language-retarded children. There is no equivalent of the speech therapist to cope with visual perception. What is needed is a 'space therapist'.

Summary (64–5)
Perception is making sense of what you see, hear and feel.
A child's perception grows along with the rest of him.
It is difficult for parents to gauge their child's perceptual development.
It is better for them to know what a child can be expected to do at certain ages.
If there is a delay in your child's development, seek advice from the child development clinic or your family doctor.
The professionals will tell you if there is a perceptual deficit and, if there is, what should be done about it.

Introduction to intelligence

Intelligence is not easy to define. It can mean 'brains', reasoning power, wit. Most of us use ourselves as the central reference point and think of others as being 'thick' if we feel that they are not as clever as we are, or as being 'too clever by half' or as 'intellectual snobs' if we are not as clever as they are. The most consoling view we can take of somebody academically successful is that, though he may be top of the class, he lacks common-sense. Intelligence is inextricably linked with memory, which stores and reproduces past events but which is dependent on the interpretation of the reality of those events by the intelligence. Parents and teachers judge a child to be intelligent or not by comparing him with other children in the family or at school. In general it is thought to be a god-given gift, an inherent capability, something which comes by chance of birth or genetics rather than something which is acquired by teaching or experience. Unless the child does not live up to adult expectations it is unlikely that his I Q will be formally ascertained, this measure of intelligence being a last resort when things have gone wrong.

66

An IQ is arrived at by carrying out an intelligence test. There are many of these available, but only one carried out by a fully qualified psychologist is of real value. Teachers, doctors and parents may do 'simple IQs', but these are at best rough tools of little value, which may positively mislead.

Intelligence is a particularly important area for parents to consider because often, when they are worried about their child, friends advise them to 'have an IQ done'. Having followed this advice, parents are little the wiser. An IQ assessment by itself is an inadequate guide to a child's future performance, but a somewhat more reliable one to his potential.

In the United Kingdom educational psychologists, as distinct from clinical ones, often do an abbreviated IQ assessment. This is a valid test as far as it goes, but it obviously does not give as detailed a view of the child's functioning as a full IQ does.

WISC-R: a general view

67 At the time of writing, the most commonly used IQ test is the Wechsler Intelligence Scale for Children, the WISC-R. The 'R' means revised version, which in 1974 replaced the original Wechsler Intelligence Scale for Children, the WISC without the 'R'. In the United Kingdom, the British Ability Scales were recently introduced. Most psychologists seem to use these as a back-up test, using part rather than the whole battery, while continuing to apply the WISC-R, which is familiar to the present generation of teachers.

The WISC-R is made up of a series of sub-tests, verbal and performance/spatial. Each sub-test is an intellectual ladder up which it is possible to scramble a certain distance. At an early age, that distance will be less than that which can be travelled when the child is older. A five-year-old is not expected to do as well in any one sub-test as an eight-year-old. Once the distance travelled along the test has been determined, then a score, a raw score, can be worked out. This, when adjusted for age, becomes the 'scaled score'. The sub-test scaled scores in each group are then amalgamated to produce a 'verbal IQ' and a 'non-verbal/performance IQ'. These two may be melded into the 'full scale IQ' and it is this final figure which may be taken as the predictor of a child's academic future or as an indication of his intellectual capacity. All things being equal and provided that nothing serious happens to the child in the way of illness, the IQ should remain constant throughout his school life. The scores obtained on the verbal, performance and full scale WISC-R IQs may be used to put a child's intellectual functioning into a specific category. An average child of average intelligence will get an average IQ score of between 90 and 109 points, a bright average child scores between 110 and 119 points, a dull or low average child between 80 and 89 points. A child scoring 120 to 129 points is rated as being of superior intelligence, while a child with 70 to 79 points is classified as being of borderline intelligence. With a score of below 70 the child is mentally retarded; a score of above 129 indicates that he is of very superior intelligence.

The cut-off levels between each category are sharply defined, so that a one-point difference may suggest that a child seems to be much more or less intelligent than in fact he is. Therefore the psychologist always comments on the results. Psychologists use IQ scores in the way a medical doctor uses a temperature reading or a blood test result, to confirm a view of the whole child. It is most important that parents and teachers realize that what the psychologist writes in the whole report is of far greater value than the IQ score by itself.

Parents must be aware that not only can the IQ score in isolation be misleading, but that the full scale may be a source of confusion unless the results of the group and sub-tests scores are considered in detail. Differences between verbal and performance scores may be hidden within a seemingly satisfactory full scale IQ and such differences may be of considerable significance. They could possibly mean that there was some underlying disease process, that there was a considerable emotional disturbance, that there was something preventing messages and stimuli from the outside world being accepted by the child, or that something was upsetting the normal processing of these messages and stimuli.

It is thought that if the verbal IQ is significantly higher than the performance IQ, then this may be related to changes in the cell structure or function of the right side of the brain. Alterations in the development of some areas, or actual damage producing an anatomical change, may sometimes underlie or be associated with abnormal psychological results. The direct scientific proof linking cell function to the results of psychological tests has not yet been firmly established. From a practical point of view, doctors will see the abnormal test results as one small piece of evidence that they need to make a diagnosis.

A similar situation arises with the differences in sub-test scores, and it is worth considering these in some detail.

Graham's parents were delighted when he made it to 'the best school in the area with a very good O-level record', a highly

academic grammar school that had recently turned comprehensive. Graham was somewhat less delighted. He was bored with classics in the first year (which became the basis of the Latin class in second and subsequent years), complained about too little enthusiasm for football and was fed up to the back teeth with two homework subjects every night. What Graham liked was going out on his BMX, or playing computer games, or fishing. Come the summer term, fishing was beginning to encroach on school time. What had been a jolly footballer in his relatively unacademic junior school had, by the second year of comprehensive school at the age of twelve years and three months, turned into a silent and morose youngster. To his parents it seemed too early for adolescent rebellion, so as a last resort they brought him to the clinic.

It took a couple of sessions alone with him to discover that there was nothing the matter with him medically; that he couldn't cope in school, really, with any subject; that his vocabulary, reading and spelling were all about the level of a nine-year-old; that he never read spontaneously – he never had and never intended to. The psychologist confirmed the doctor's impression that Graham's IQ was in the upper 80s.

Fortunately his father, an absolutely top-notch electrician, was at this time considering an offer of a job in East Anglia. The family decided to move and Graham benefited by a face-saving transfer to a well-established comprehensive school where his ability range was fully catered for.

WISC-R verbal sub-tests

68 The first of the verbal sub-tests, *information*, aims to discover the extent of the child's general knowledge. For a child under eight it starts by asking how many ears he has; up to twenty-nine questions of increasing sophistication follow, for instance one about the significance of 5 November (in the United Kingdom) or 4 July (in the United States). Children who do badly in this sub-test may have recently arrived in the country where the test is being taken, or they may not have attended school regularly, or while in school they may have been absorbed in a private imaginary world, or (for the older ones) they may have made little progress with reading for information. Obviously a degree of deafness may force a child into that private world and make it seem that he is lacking in intellectual capacity because of inadequate information. Teachers see success in this sub-test as definitely related to schooling, on the grounds that general information, clearly and briefly stated as demanded by the sub-test, is often acquired and more often articulated succinctly in schools. A capacious memory for fact, as distinct from ability to reason from fact, underpins success.

The second sub-test, *similarities*, will be familiar to teachers from 'main idea' exercises, which often come under the heading of 'study skills' or 'reading for learning'. The teacher, or the appropriate text, gives lists of related items, such as cups, saucers, plates and jugs; the pupil has to state that, collectively, they are crockery. Arguably, the longer the list the easier the identification (and the more time for thinking of the appropriate wording). In the classroom the next step is to look for more precise definitions; tulips, daffodils, hyacinths and crocuses are not just flowers, but spring flowers. In the WISC-R sub-test the child is given, at any one time, only two items which have to be linked by their descent from a shared category. A maximum of seventeen pairs of words may be considered.

Difficulty in word-finding [90] can scupper success in this sub-test, just as difficulty with verbal concept formation can. A number of books in common use in schools have exercises to foster ability for categorization. In primary schools these exercises concern, for instance, modes of transport: what is used for water transport as distinct from air transport. In secondary schools the periodic table of chemical elements or the classification of plants shows the relationship between items and provides the framework in which to remember them. Teachers are well aware that the ability to categorize is an aid not only to understanding but also to memory.

Patrick was distinctly worried about himself. He wanted to take a few science O-levels and was clearly very well taught in school. As he explained, he knew what he had to learn and learnt it, but it somehow never seemed enough. His teachers boomed 'only connect'; he had no idea what they meant. No, he didn't like reading, he had never read for fun. He had quite a profitable sideline in reconstructing bicycles and this took up all his spare time. Did he listen to spoken-word programmes on the radio while working on the bikes? No, not at all, he was into heavy metal.

His IQ scores provided the answer: an IQ that would

theoretically stretch to O-levels took a very, very deep dip on the information sub-test. No wonder such information as he had floated in a limbo of unconnected fact.

Since he wasn't going to change his habits at this stage he was advised to listen to serious spoken-word programmes at every opportunity.

If ever a bombshell walked into the clinic it was Gillie. Aged eight, she was a brilliant red-head with a sweet smile. We all gaped, and the teacher had unworthy thoughts about the need for reading if a girl looked like that.

In fact Gillie was an extremely nice little girl, good-mannered and demure. But she could not read, either continuous prose, or single words by word recognition or phonic build-up. Her physical coordination and her receptive vocabulary for single words was extremely good, and so was her memory for instructions as long as the objects for acting out the instructions were in front of her. She could barely tackle spelling, she formed letters in a haphazard way, she placed words at random on the page and she had not the remotest idea what a rhyme was although she remembered, imperfectly, several nursery rhymes.

The clinical psychologist's report came through: within an IQ generally in the average range, the score for similarities was at precipice depth. No wonder she could not categorize by sound, or by anything else. Suggestions were made about learning-by-doing, and categorizing activities for home and school were listed. It was difficult to imagine how patternless the world must seem to her.

The third sub-test reduces many children and a significant propor-tion of adults to panic. It is concerned with *arithmetic*, and it is timed, the maximum allowance per question being thirty seconds. Most of the questions are orally presented, and none of them are straight sums of the 'ten, take away four, leaves ... what?' variety. Most of them are tiny 'number stories'; for instance: 'A farmer had fourteen sheep and he sold five. How many did he have left?' In this way the sum is embedded in verbal distractors; if the child is to cope with the question, the story must be heard accurately, understood, held in mind while the required sum is extracted, the operation (or series of them) decided on and executed, and the final answer given orally.

Success in this sub-test depends on not panicking, on a good auditory memory [73], on understanding not only the mathematical ideas embedded in the text but also mathematical terms like 'equally' or 'dozen', as well as sheer computational ability. Obviously, if this kind of mind-sharpening exercise has been done frequently in school the practice effect carries over into the test also, not least because familiarity often dispels panic.

If the child does badly in this sub-test, consider also his scores on the 'digit span' [68] and 'coding" [69] sub-tests. If all three are low, is it because he is particularly distractable? If the answer is 'yes', consider his restlessness further. The paragraphs on hyperkinesis [134] and stress [128] may be relevant.

If, on the other hand, the questions are answered correctly but outside the specified time limits, more inquiries are in order. Is the child very slow at all information-processing? The British Ability Scales sub test for this will prove illuminating. Is he a 'belt and braces' lad who double- and triple-checks everything? Is he unable to do sums in his head because he has seldom been asked to? Can he do them on paper or with a calculator?

The *vocabulary* sub-test consists of the examiner saying a word and inviting the child to give its meaning. It starts off, apparently harmlessly, with 'bike' (though a child under eight might have trouble in describing its essential characteristics) and rapidly escalates the difficulty far beyond the first or second thousand words most commonly found in print. The width of a child's experience and the level of language used to discuss them affect success. The reliability of his memory and the quality of his education will also contribute to success in this sub-test by extending his intellectual capacity.

A shortfall in this area can have quite startling results for an older child. Andrew was sixteen when first seen in the clinic, with a history of epilepsy and an IQ in the bright average range except for a plummeting score for vocabulary. He had been very successful in public examinations (O-levels) in maths and chemistry and was preparing for more exams in subjects where language plays a greater part. His difficulty was in his failure to understand the textbooks he was meant to be working from, in physics as much as in history, or the wording of the questions. By the time he had puzzled out the meaning of an exam question he had little time left to answer it. The example he gave was 'the kingdom of the fox', bewildering when books and teachers had referred to 'the habitat of the fox'. He was teaching himself physics by re-telling, on paper and in his own words, the salient features of the topics on the syllabus. This worked well, for that was how he had coped with chemistry, but was very slow; he had only five months in which to do the same for biology, geography, history, economics and English. School, which had known for several years about his problem, offered no help. Andrew was, understandably, a very worried and unhappy young man, for he realized how much slower he was than his peers at accumulating facts and forming concepts.

The next sub-test, *comprehension*, is about problem-solving. The truant with his wits about him usually shines in this test, designed to discover how far the subject is aware of the practical and moral demands of daily living. The fourteen questions start with something simple and straightforward, like what to do if you cut your thumb ('Suck it' or 'Go to Mum' are not the best replies); there is one about how to cope with a train approaching an obstacle on the line, where a joky response is not in order. Children fall down on this sub-test if their answers are too specific. For instance, one question asks what to do if, on being sent to buy bread, there turns out to be none in the shop. A particular child, knowing that in his immediate neighbourhood the next bread shop is across a busy road he is not allowed to cross alone, may reply reasonably: 'I'd go back home and tell Mum.' This will not earn full marks unless the reason for his reply is given and the rider is added, 'but of course someone would have to go to another shop to buy some'. Not all children feel sufficiently communicative, or have the presence of mind, to enlarge their replies until they arrive at what is the best response for all cases (that is, to take the general view) as opposed to the best response in their own particular circumstances. Since the questions in this sub-test involve judgement of particular circumstances, longer and more elaborate replies are in order. These will give an idea, in the first place, of how far a child is aware of social conventions; second, how independent and self-confident he may be; and third, what attitudes he has absorbed, or is fighting against, from his family's view of life.

The last verbal sub-test is called *digit span*. It is a test of auditory sequential memory [73], and two aspects are examined:

1. Straight capacity of sequential memory is assessed by the tester saying digits at one-second intervals with the subject immediately repeating them. Three digits are presented in the first instance, and the maximum possible sequence is one of nine digits. There is no penalty for repeating the digits as whole numbers, as in 'forty-two thousand six-hundred and fifty-seven' as distinct from 'four-two-six-five-seven'.

2. Flexibility of memory is assessed by the tester saying the digits at one-second intervals and asking the subject to repeat them in reverse order. If the tester says 'two-five-seven-four', the correct response is 'four-seven-five-two'. The trials start with two digits and can be extended to eight.

Arguably a few children used to the French way with telephone numbers – grouping them in pairs: 'forty-two, sixty-five, seven' – should shine in this test. In other words, putting random numbers into a pattern is a potent aid to remembering them. This is particularly useful in the 'digits in reverse order' section of the test, which calls for the numbers to be held in mind long enough for them to be re-strung into a new pattern, and the new pattern to be voiced.

Ability in this sub-test relates closely to schooling: a good memory for digits carries over into a good memory for instructions [31]; it helps the formation of full sentences and it allows the phonic approach to reading and spelling to be used with a good chance of success. Consider a word like 'continual': four syllables, four different vowels each clearly heard; how are they to be assembled in the right order and inserted between the equally audible consonants unless the whole word can be correctly enunciated, broken into its syllables repeatedly, rapidly and often internally (that is, 'sounded in your head') until the whole is written down? An inadequate auditory sequential memory sabotages this process. But why should it be inadequate? Most often because of difficulties with listening [31] or stress [128].

WISC-R performance sub-tests

The performance half of the WISC-R test consists of five timed sub-tests. Bonus points may be gained for completing each task rapidly, and all tasks can be performed in complete silence on the part of the child being tested. Adequate visual acuity and visual perception (the inferential process which makes sense of the visual stimuli impinging on

69

the eyes) are needed for all the sub-tests, and some also call for good hand–eye coordination.

Picture completion is the greatest fun. The child is presented with the drawing of a familiar object from which one indispensable component has been omitted, for instance one leg of a chair. The tester asks, 'What is missing in this picture?' and the child answers either verbally or by pointing. This test is reminiscent of what teachers call 'cloze exercises' – that is paragraphs or complete stories from which words have been deleted and the pupil has to insert the missing words. In a verbal task there is of course scope for variation: a girl may be described as thin, slender, slim, lean or skinny without significantly altering the total impact of the passage. But a drawing of an insect is seriously at fault if the antennae have been omitted. In other words, the child has to distinguish the features of prime importance from secondary ones.

Success in this test probably depends on the child being in the habit of looking at objects attentively and enumerating, at least to himself, their constituent features. For instance, a clock face, as long as it isn't a digital clock, must have two hands (some have a third one), twelve signs for the hours (though some clocks have twenty-four) and additional signs for the minutes. If a child has at some time in the past articulated this description, or discussed the features of various types of clock face with a better-informed mentor, he has a very good chance of always recognizing a clock face and knowing which parts are missing. In short, earlier language experience, allied to observation of a wide variety of objects and a good visual memory for them, leads to success in this sub-test.

Picture arrangement is the second of the WISC-R sub-tests and examines sequencing ability. The tester lays a number of representational pictures in front of the child. As laid down in random order they make no sequential sense; they don't 'tell a story that makes sense'. The child is invited to rearrange them so that they do. A minimum of four and a maximum of six cards are used in any one of seven sequences. In four of these sequences alternative arrangements, leading to somewhat different story lines, are credited – up to a point. If the child lays down the cards so that the story starts from the right rather than, conventionally, from the left, points are obtained as long as the sequence is coherent.

For this test the child must first understand what the individual pictures convey, what event in a story or episode in a series of events the picture represents or could represent. In this respect the sub-test is reminiscent of the vocabulary sub-test in the verbal part of the WISC-

R, where the meaning, or more than one meaning, of a word is sought. Then the separate pictures have to be fitted into a sequential pattern of recognized behaviour, 'a story that makes sense', much in the way that responses in the comprehension sub-test are expected to echo accepted behaviour. In short, several potential stories have to be held in mind and compared while the starting-point of the story and the optimum consequential steps are decided upon. The complication here is the sequence of events. You can't weigh the ingredients for a cake after it has been put in the oven. A verbal gloss, however eloquent, will achieve few points, although it may show that the child is a divergent rather than a convergent thinker, an important point if an individual programme of tuition, tailored to his particular strengths, is being planned.

In contrast to the digit span sub-test, which tests sequential memory for abstract information orally presented, this test assesses ability to sequence large units of meaning, visually presented. Children with extensive experience of both hearing and telling stories, and of explanations giving cause and effect, are likely to do better at this. Familiarity with comic strips with narrative rather than mainly joke content also helps. Heretical as it may sound, *Asterix* and *Tintin* are preferable to *Beano*.

Block design is the most abstract of the sub-tests. A child of eight or over is shown a design on a card and is given red and white cubes to reproduce the design with. Having done this, he is shown the next card which has a design of increasing difficulty. Each step is harder and the number of cubes to be used increases from four to nine.

This sub-test calls for ability to take apart a design into its component parts and then re-synthesize it using the blocks. Thus visual perception and organization are tested, in the same way – but more elaborately – as auditory discrimination and organization are tested [103], as well as the ability to recognize and re-create concepts which it is difficult to label verbally. If the child fails in this sub-test, the important question to ask is: Is the cause of the failure an inability to identify the particular design, or the inability to reproduce it? In cases of doubt, clinical psychologists have access to other tests which can elucidate the point. The manner of tackling each successive task is also important; is the child using random trial and error or a more considered strategy? The tasks in this sub-test are, in their upper limits, certainly more difficult than the various multicoloured 'tile design' toys familiar from nursery and infant classes. However, pleasure and competence in playing with these should help towards success with the block design sub-test.

Object assembly is another sub-test which is great fun. It consists of four jig-saws which have to be put together, one at a time and in the normal way, to form frequently-seen objects. The maximum number of pieces used is eight, making this sub-test similar to the large, simple wooden jig-saws of, perhaps, a horse or steam engine that very young children enjoy. However, the toy jig-saws have a recessed outline of the finished object, so that a recognizable silhouette can guide the child's understanding of the relationships of the parts to the whole. The sub-test materials offer no such guide. Further, the pieces are not necessarily immediately recognizable. The child has to form a hypothetical pattern, hold it in mind long enough to compare the partly assembled pieces against it, and if necessary start again. As the assembling of pieces progresses, the remaining pieces and their orientation become more readily identifiable. So perception and organization are again involved, as in the block design sub-test, only this time the whole and the parts can be easily labelled with words from the child's normal vocabulary. Obviously, visuo-motor control also plays an important part, particularly in the sensory feedback derived from handling the pieces. If the child fails, several questions need to be asked. Is the failure due to imperfect motor control? Is the visual feedback below par? Is the child unable to hypothesize on the identity of any single piece? If so, can he not extrapolate from that the nature of the whole object? In the last instance, visual memory for objects seen in the daily welter may be at fault.

Coding, the last sub-test of the WISC-R, is exactly what its name implies. The child is asked to copy symbols which are paired with another set of symbols set out in the key placed at the top of the form on which the test is done. Children under eight have a key with five symbols and the older ones have nine. The test should be done in red pencil or red pen, with no rubbing-out. This sub-test examines the ability to use newly acquired information quickly and precisely. It is another look at hand–eye co-ordination, with considerable application to hand-writing and spelling. Attention and pertinacity in accomplishing a task are also tested.

It had been noted over a long period that many children with reading and spelling difficulties have low scores on this sub-test. It was suggested that the reason for this might be that the test was the last of the whole batch and consequently the child was tired. A controlled experiment was carried out, asking children to do this sub-test first. It made no difference to the level of scores or the incidence of low ones.

During the same period, other independent research was done which revealed low scores on this subject to be associated with diffuse changes in the electroencephalogram [121].

The importance of the WISC-R

You will have noticed that some sub-tests of the WISC-R can be **70** grouped according to the ability they examine. One threesome, consisting of 'digit span', 'picture arrangement' and 'coding', examines sequencing ability, but different aspects of it. 'Digit span' focuses on short-term memory for sequences of abstract material which has only been heard. 'Picture arrangement' deals with visually presented material that has to be placed in a coherent story sequence; there is no load on short-term memory, for the pictures stay put. However, long-term memory is called on in the interpretation of the individual pictures as parts of logical sequences of events recognized from the child's past experience. (Here it also links with the 'comprehension' sub-test.) 'Coding' is back to short-term memory for sequences of abstract symbols, but visual this time, although there is nothing against the child labelling them verbally to himself; if he does so silently no one is any the wiser, short of direct questioning. Labelling the abstract symbols may well speed up his performance, which also calls upon visuo-motor coordination, which in turn is engaged in a repetitive sequence of tasks.

If a child does badly on all these three sub-tests, the chances are that he will have trouble with all sequences: days, months, the alphabet, telephone numbers, spelling, learning anything by heart, remembering instructions, telling or re-telling stories. Life for him will be significantly less ordered and predictable than for the average child.

Another linked threesome consists of 'block design', 'object assembly' and 'coding'. All three call for visuo-motor coordination: information obtained through the eyes programmes the movement of the hands and fingers. If in the first two, 'block design' and 'object assembly', a child 'lets the hands do the thinking', that is, assembles the pattern and objects on a trial-and-error basis, it suggests that visual information is inadequately processed. It is evident that two distinct ways of processing visual stimuli are called for: 'block design' starts with an abstract whole, breaks it down into its component parts and reassembles it. 'Object assembly' starts with perhaps meaningless and therefore abstract parts: these have to be assembled into a recognizable whole which will have its echo in the child's long-term memory. Consider a child examining pieces of a jig-saw that he doesn't recognize until he comes upon one that he knows represents an elephant's trunk. He remembers what an elephant looks like. Once he has reached this stage, the task of assembling the elephant (the child knows he is looking for tusks, large ears, huge body, small tail and four legs) goes much faster, the only possible stumbling-block being the precise position of the pieces for the legs and parts of the huge body, assuming that has been divided into several pieces. At this stage the orientation of the particular pieces is being considered, a process that is particularly important in the 'block design' sub-test. 'Coding' finally demands good visuo-motor organization; there is no reasoning involved, and good short-term memory speeds up performance. Performance in the 'coding' sub-test has direct bearing on handwriting and spelling.

If you consider the WISC-R as the sum of its constituent sub-tests you may see these not only as measuring a cluster of faculties with a given amount of overlap. There is another important link between all of them: every one involves an aspect of memory. 'Information', 'similarities', 'vocabulary', 'comprehension' and 'picture arrangement' are dependent on memory for meaning; as a slight variation, in 'object assembly' the memory is visual. 'Digit span' calls for short-term auditory sequential memory, and in its second half (digits backwards) an operational demand is added; arithmetic calls for the same short-term auditory operational memory. 'Block design' and 'coding' are underpinned by short-term visual operational memory, while 'picture completion' requires long-term visual memory.

There is a further aspect of individual sub-test scores that is important. Suppose the child has broadly consistent scores for most of them except for a dramatic dip in one or two. The results for education can be far-reaching, as has been explained in section 68. But medically the dip can also be significant. The doctor's observation of the child may have led to suspicions of organic damage. The clinical psychologist is called in to administer, in the first place, the WISC-R in order either to scotch the suspicion or to confirm it; if the latter is the case she will also provide information about its severity and impairing effect. The clinical psychologist's repertoire includes a number of tests, other than the WISC-R, to pinpoint and assess organic damage.

So remember that parental expectation aroused by an IQ score must be tempered by the psychologist's report. Have sympathy with any psychologist who may be reluctant to put a precise figure on your child's intelligence. Firstly, she may regard her own findings with some suspicion and feel that they may not be so precise as a bald numerical score might suggest. Secondly, she may be afraid that you will get the wrong end of the stick and jump to the conclusion that just because your child has a high full-scale WISC-R score he is necessarily going to achieve wonders at school. If he is bright and distractable he is likely to do very well in the WISC-R (the one-to-one attention is most flattering) but badly in school. If he is unable to organize himself, he may still do very well in the limited structured tasks of the sub-tests but be quite unable to cope with wider assignments (such as writing appraisals, essays, compiling a thematic topic folder) where success depends on selecting and presenting a small range of relevant material extracted from a much wider pool of information.

The verbal IQ holds one further confusion for parents. Though it tests a child's potential to communicate, the results do not always seem to tally with those of a speech therapist. You may get an average verbal IQ and a speech therapist's report that the child's language is delayed. Muddling, to say the least. The speech therapists and the psychologists are testing different things. The therapist is concerned with language as a flowing stream of words. She looks to find words strung together in the right context, in the right order, with correct expression and understanding, and of a complexity and maturity appropriate to the child's age. She will also test listening skills, and speed of reception and production. Her language is in the normal context of the playground and the home. The 'microscope' she uses is of a higher power than that of the psychologist. She is more sensitive to variations from the normal which may presage deviations from the normal. It may take her several sessions with the child to determine exactly what is wrong; she may want to come into the classroom to listen to the child in a normal setting, and then go home to play back tape recordings of his language in an effort to analyse what is going on. So you have to put together both the therapist's and the psychologist's reports. If they seem at variance, ask both of them, 'Why the difference?'

An example may clarify the difference between the speech therapist's estimate of language and the psychologist's measurements of it for the WISC-R.

In a particular sub-test, one of the sixteen possible questions asked is: 'In what way are an apple and a banana alike?' A little girl of seven replied that both had skins and under the skin they were both white, and both grew on trees, and she ate them raw or cooked, and they were jolly good for picnics or snacks or packed lunches. Fair enough, you would think, and the speech therapist and the child's parents thought so too. But not the psychologist, who was looking for the plain statement that both apples and bananas are fruit. In this sub-test the psychologist was looking for the child's ability to categorize and find names for the categories. In general, she is looking for the child's use of language as a cognitive tool and an aid to making sense of experience. The speech therapist was looking for communicative ability, the response to experience and the ability to report it.

If a child has a low I Q, this may account for his late acquisition of literacy, but not always. It is possible to have a low I Q plus a delay in language development, the two together producing a state of affairs that suggests that only special schooling will help. If, however, the language delay is recognized and tackled, the outcome may surprise everyone. It is not enough to classify a child as having 'poor global intelligence' and assume that no further investigation is necessary. Quite apart from any medical condition which might be causing this, there may be a concomitant language problem. Do not be content with a diagnosis of a broad generality, such as 'slow learner', 'mild educational difficulties' or whatever the up-to-date phrase may be. In such cases it is important to find out why this state of affairs exists, because it may be treatable by other than teaching techniques.

There is one more snag: poor readers do not become familiar with the language of books as do those children whose noses are always stuck into literature. The vocabulary and information sub-tests depend increasingly on reading as junior school gives way to secondary, so a verbal I Q may drop off in later childhood because more time is spent *doing* than *reading*.

Lastly, though IQs may be seen as predictive, there is value in repeating them if the child's performance is declining. Marked changes in I Q may be related to disease, so do not blame an obvious change in scores on 'not trying' – the child may be ill.

Howard came to the clinic sporting a neat chinstrap beard, to emphasize that, at just eighteen, he was definitely in his last year of school and raring to go on to higher education. He was quite sure he would be studying chemistry. But, much to his puzzlement, he had twice failed O-level chemistry, the only public examination he had tried to do, necessary for his entry to higher education. He did, or rather tried to do, the usual tests of oral reading, silent reading comprehension and spelling suitable for chronological age, and came out as barely literate:

his mechanical reading was comparable with that of a nine-year-old, his silent reading had not developed at all, his spelling was weaker still.

When the reasons for doubting entry to higher education were explained to him he indignantly produced, like a rabbit out of a hat, a much-handled piece of paper. This was a psychologist's report of a WISC test done when he was nine. At the time his IQ was comfortably in the superior range, quite adequate for entry to university, although the psychologist had noted that he was lagging behind with reading and spelling.

It was suggested that the persistent reading delay had weakened his chances of higher education. He counterclaimed that his native intelligence was sufficient to overcome the lack of reading. After some to-ing and fro-ing, he insisted on having his IQ re-tested. It came out as average.

Moral: If you don't use it, you lose it.

Summary (66–70)

Only a qualified psychologist can administer a proper IQ test.

The most common IQ test is the WISC-R; it is divided into sub-tests. These measure the ability to communicate, to think things out for oneself, and some aspects of memory.

Big differences between the sub-test scores may indicate some underlying disturbance.

The psychologist's report is as important as the scores themselves.

An IQ score is a guide to school potential and has to be put in the context of the child's health, personality and background.

School performance is influenced more by the worst scores in the IQ than the best.

Illness can change an IQ; if a child cannot read, some IQ scores will drop.

Long-term memories

It is not known just how memory works, or exactly where it is to be found. It develops hand-in-hand with the physiological growth of the brain. It is essential to the learning, remembering and forgetting processes. There are two sorts of memory: long-term and short-term. Long-term memory is long-lasting and durable. It holds material learnt and

71

the meaning of that material. It may be subdivided into *semantic* and *episodic* fractions.

Semantic memory enables us to solve crossword puzzles. It holds facts which may be shared by all of us and is capable of answering questions like: 'Who discovered America?', or 'Who wrote *Hamlet*?'

Episodic memory is personal. It holds information about our very own experiences. It can answer questions like: 'What did I do yesterday morning?', or 'What colour was the wallpaper in my first bedroom?'. Loss of this episodic/personal memory is what most of us understand when we hear that someone is suffering from loss of memory, has been found wandering and cannot recall anything about himself. Items held in these long-term memories are extracted, dusted down, re-examined; the very fact of recalling and rehearsing them serves to fix them more firmly in long-term memory. Visual, auditory and other experiences can be stored.

Short-term memories

72 Short-term memory is a temporary storage system. It plays an important part in learning and language comprehension. It holds items for short periods only, during which they may become organized in order to be fixed in the long-term memory, especially if the items are repeated. The organization will amount to scanning a newly encountered stimulus for some feature or segment which relates to a similar one held in the long-term memory. A very crude example: when we see for the first time the blue-and-white double-decker buses in Athens we may relate them to red, yellow or multicoloured double-decker buses in London and elsewhere. Without such an echo the new stimulus lacks meaning. It is that much more difficult for it to enter long-term memory.

For purposes of reading and writing, the important feature of short-term memory is that it holds the order or sequence in which items are presented. It is therefore subdivided into auditory and visual sequential memories.

Auditory and visual sequential memory

73 The auditory short-term memory may respond to material via speech. Even when looking at written material we may mouth it quietly to ourselves to activate this system. If the radio is blaring at the same time, this is difficult to do.

The visual sequential memory is weaker than the auditory. It holds sequences of shapes seen. If the shapes cannot be coded into sounds, as letters can, for example, then that background radio does not make much difference; it does not muddle the sequencing capability.

Both speech therapists and psychologists test short-term memories [102, 70], presenting auditory and visual sequences to a child and asking him to repeat them immediately. From the results they can say whether a child's short-term memory is as could be expected for his age or not.

An easy, but not scientifically accurate, way of thinking about these short-term memories is to regard them as the mind's ears and eyes. The speech therapist may ask the child to repeat a series of digits, saying, for example, 'one-five-nine-four'. The child has to hold them in his mind's ear long enough to be able to repeat them back to her in the right order. The same thing happens with speech sounds. If the child has a poor short-term auditory memory, he will forget what has been said in the middle of a long sentence. This happens to children with poor listening skills resulting from ear infections in early life [31]. Understanding is lost because the poor short-term memory does not record the incoming information and does not hold it in the mind's ear.

The same may happen with sequences of shapes seen, except that these must be held in the mind's eye rather than in the ear. However, if the shapes are letters, they have phonic qualities and the child may use sub-vocal speech to process them. He calls in the auditory short-term memory to bolster his poor short-term visual memory. Children with poor short-term visual sequential memories can be seen to mouth words as they try to read them, using slow phonic analysis to identify each word. This hinders learning and visual recall so that their spelling is faulty, especially in English which, until you have learnt the rules, is illogical when it comes to relating speech sounds to spelling. Phonic capability alone is a poor prop to correct orthography.

Those unfortunate children who have *both* short-term memories at fault are in a disastrous situation. They have grave difficulty in holding in mind any stimulus long enough to process it into long-term memory. As a result, long-term memory is the poorer and this in turn makes the organizing function of short-term memory that much less effective. The only (partial) way out of this situation is to present these children with information that relates to their immediate needs, pleasures and distresses and, by patient conversation accompanying action, try to build routines which will see them through concrete daily tasks. Symbolic information from books, teachers talking in school, even TV, will for the most part just wash over them like water off a duck's back.

Angela was a pretty little dark-haired girl, the middle one of three children, the eldest being a very clever sister and the youngest 'a real boy'. She had been deaf until the age of three and a half, when her adenoids had been removed, grommets inserted and no other treatment suggested.

School was fairly disastrous from the start, and since she was clearly bright it was assumed that she was being exceptionally self-willed and defiant, as well as aggressive towards the other children. Her parents, who saw her as a failure, had had her under psychoanalysis for three years, with no beneficial results. When seen at the clinic at the age of nine years and six months, she was very anxious and made efforts to keep up a good front. Her audiogram was fine, but her vocabulary, memory for instructions and auditory sequential memory were abysmal. In a reading test she could mouth print very competently, but in no way understand what she had just read. If, encouraged by school and at home, she read to herself, she did it aloud and – unsurprisingly – remembered little of it.

What could be done? At this late stage the speech therapist's contribution – which would have made all the difference at the age of three and a half – would be marginal. Advice was offered on 'chunking' [31, 37]; it was suggested that she should be helped to invent and sketch (for she drew very well) mnemonics, diagrams, use lists, etc. For future advanced work (an academic school was not advised) cognitive maps and the analytic study of texts would help, but immediately she needed to be given her head with activities she enjoyed and was good at (drawing, cooking, Brownies) to regain her self-confidence.

His mother had not been well towards the end of the pregnancy; Donald had been born slowly as the labour was long. He was a bit blue on arrival because of too little oxygen, but rapidly recovered and was not kept in intensive care. He was a restless baby, but passed his milestones of walking and talking sentences at the right times. As he got older it was noticed that he had difficulty in pronouncing long words; the family used to think some of his muddles were rather funny.

He did all right at school at first; he was friendly and

energetic without being rowdy. He was, in fact, something of a conformer, sticking rigidly to 'the rules of the school'.

However, by the time he was seven he was obviously having some difficulty in learning to read and was very slow to cope with reading aloud. If he had to do this in class, the rest of the children used to mock him. His spelling was very poor. His mother said that he would learn words by writing them out several times and would know them the next morning, only to forget them by the next week.

When seen in the clinic at the age of ten he was obviously under considerable stress. He looked tense and anxious, had a stomach-ache which had come on that morning (but which wore off when he found that we were not going to eat him) and wanted to know whether he had got each item right before he moved on to the next. 'Did I get it right?' was his constant query.

His IQ showed him to be of bright average intelligence [67] though he scored very badly in the 'coding' sub-test [69]. The speech therapist found that he had normal language and good listening skills, but that he had a very poor visual sequential memory.

When he had to read aloud in the Neale test [165] he was very slow. He could be seen to mouth words to himself before he risked saying them. However, he was very accurate and made no mistakes in comprehension. He understood exactly what he had read. His scores, apart from those for speed, were normal for his age and intelligence. He read silently much more efficiently and with good understanding.

His spelling was a phonic disaster. Words were written exactly as they sounded (he spelt 'peculiar' 'perquler') and the book of compositions which he showed us was full of crossings-out. Words would be re-spelt, corrected and rewritten so that the end result was a very short piece of work covered in corrections. At the bottom of most pieces of work, the teacher had written 'more care with spelling', followed by a list of words for him to learn.

His pattern of performance was one that was all too familiar to the clinic staff.

What is the cause of the poor short-term visual sequential memory? There is some dispute about this. Medical examination reveals that such children have difficulty doing things in sequence: they are better at cross-country running than table tennis. They may be travel-sick. They cannot hold the order of things seen in their mind's eye. Electroencephalograms [121] are usually normal. There are no signs of damage to the cerebral hemispheres. There is a considerable body of opinion which regards this difficulty as being one of sequencing, owing to a cerebellar weakness of coordination [59]. The problem seems to be not so much one of memory as one of patterning a programme for instant use. There is some suggestion that the condition might respond to medication, but evidence for this is not convincing. Unfortunately the cerebellum is difficult to investigate, hidden as it is under the main brain.

In the long term, children such as Donald do quite well in life provided that their confidence and self-esteem have not been destroyed by constant failure to write satisfactory compositions.

Topographical agnosia

74 There is an uncommon form of memory-loss sometimes seen among children with learning disabilities. This is the inability to remember their bearings. They cannot find their way about, even in places with which they could be expected to be familiar. They get lost outside their own front door. They may also have difficulty with spatial orientation but it may be much more specific than that.

It is thought that there is some fault or delay in development of the posterior portions of the parietal lobes of the cerebral cortex [55, 56; Figure 4]. There may be two components:

1. An inability to cope with the spatial layout of a route, that is, inefficient map-reading.
2. A faulty memory for the buildings or features which make up the landmarks of the route.

It seems likely that in these cases the right half of the brain is more important than the left.

Vicky was a nice girl of twelve, mad keen on riding and far less keen on school. She was bad at geography, poor at geometry and not much use at spelling. She had to be taken to school by her father, even though the school was only two streets away in the same block. The parents recognized that she was not a 'school refuser', because they also had to take her to the riding stables which were in the same block but in the opposite direction. She could never find her way to either establishment and always had to be escorted.

Activities with Scouts or Guides, orienteering, and – increasingly used in schools – computer programs on map-reading combine to diminish embarrassment caused by this quirky disability.

Improvement?

Over the years the clinic at which the authors work has sent out suggestions, devised mostly by the speech therapists, for improving memory generally and principally auditory memory. It cannot honestly be said that the results have been encouraging. By and large children, like adults, remember best what they want to remember, and the larger the unit the better; that is, a child will remember a complete sentence of four to ten words, or its contents, more reliably than he will remember four to ten disparate words. Nothing new in that. To which can be added these crumbs of comfort:

1. Certainly the alleviation of disease, and especially anxiety and clinical depression, improves the sufferer's memory all round [128, 130].

2. Enabling a child to hear better, perhaps by the insertion of grommets, improves his auditory memory, possibly because once he can hear more and more clearly, there is more for the memory to latch on to [31, 32].

3. In the case of children with histories of early hearing loss [31], if instructions are 'chunked' the child finds it easier to listen and follow them. Conversely, continuous speech with subordinate clauses is much harder. Compare the following passages:

The old lady with the little girl, who was wearing a blue coat, was telling the bus queue how they had been waiting for half an hour.

There was a queue at the bus stop. At the head were an old lady and a little girl. The little girl was wearing a blue coat. They had been waiting for the bus for half an hour. The old lady was telling the bus queue about the long wait.

4. With maturation, visual sequential memory often improves [73].

5. Handwriting proficiency is closely linked with memory for spelling [192].

6. By the same token, joining eye, ear and hand (for movement and for feeling textures and shapes of letters) reinforces memory for the shape of words and the sequence of letters making them up [168].

7. Mnemonics can help ('Richard Of York Gave Battle In Vain' for the colours of the spectrum), often bringing in another type of stimulus (for example, a cartoon to be copied with a caption: 'We're back where we were yesterday').

8. Putting a particular item of information into as many contexts of related information (classifying in several ways) helps.

9. Lists, timetables, diaries; transferring information from books or lectures on to diagrams, charts, cognitive maps (for instance, the periodic table) – all these are helpful. For secondary school texts, analysing them for the features related to the particular text type is a hopeful new technique.

Just plain repetition of, say, the multiplication tables does not work. Meaning, that is, by working out the sums or a catchy tune, does.

Summary (71–5)

There are two types of memory: long- and short-term.

Long-term memory lasts for years, and may be divided into two: a memory for facts which are shared with other people; and a memory for what has happened to oneself, which is personal.

Short-term memory is a temporary storage system.

Short-term memory has two important components in relation to reading and spelling: auditory and visual sequential memory.

With the auditory sequential memory, the order in which sounds are heard is held while being recognized as a word.

A weak auditory sequential memory may be caused by ear disease.

Poor listening skills, poor understanding of what is said, and poor spelling result.

With the visual sequential memory, the order in which shapes are seen is held while being recognized as a word.

A weak visual sequential memory causes slow reading, poor spelling and poor elementary mathematics.

Topographical agnosia is a loss of memory for where one is; it is rare.

Chapter Eight
Agility and Clumsiness

Normal motor development

In the old days when we had to walk everywhere, the milestone told us how far we had come, each one passed cheering us on the way. For the child travelling the road from infancy to maturity, the milestones are the indicators of achievements in time, rather than distance. Easily recognizable stages of development are called 'milestones' by the doctors. They are not so clear-cut as those little white markers by the main road. Each medical milestone indicates what the average child can be expected to be doing at a certain age. There is some variation within the bounds of normality. When the clock strikes midnight on the twenty-eighth day of your child's life, do not get in a fuss if he has not passed the milestone labelled 'four weeks'. You must take the following information as a rough guide and not as a strict ruling.

At first, the very young baby has difficulty in fastening on to the nipple to feed, so milk may dribble out of the corner of his mouth. By about the fifth month, his mouth movements are under better control and he can put his lips to the rim of a cup well enough to get a drink from it. At six months, he starts to chew and can get hold of things, and he will hang on to the bottle at feed-time. To begin with, your baby waves both his arms about indiscriminately. By the time he is nine months old, one hand leads when he stretches for a toy, which he then passes from hand to hand in equal exploration. Do not bother which hand he takes your offerings with; let him choose for himself. At a year, he is on the move, bottom up in the air, using all four limbs to get about. If you want him to walk, you have to give him a helping hand. He is coy, but if you ask nicely he may give you a kiss; Adam's first response to Eve's apple. When he points at what he wants, you may notice a preference for one hand beginning to show. He will have learnt to play pat-a-cake and he may be able to pick up small things with his forefinger and thumb.

Three months later he can get himself upright and may walk without help. Stopping is a problem and turning corners impossible.

He throws things out of his cot, but if you encourage him to throw something when he is standing, he will probably fall over. Put on his shoes and he will take them off.

At eighteen months he is up and down stairs, but has to hold on to the rail. He can climb a bit, he can jump with both feet at once. He throws a ball without falling over. He may be copying you doing the housework. He can sit on a chair. Give him a book and he will turn pages in a bunch. His hand preference is more obvious and you should have a pretty good idea whether he is right- or left-handed. He will still use both hands to play with toys. Gloves, socks and zips are taken off or undone.

By his second birthday he goes downstairs, both feet on each tread together, still holding the banister. He may walk backwards if you show him how. He can kick a ball without walking into it, though this depends on opportunity. Give him a garden and an older brother as a model, and you may have an embryo Liverpool striker in the family. You should know for sure now whether he is right- or left-handed. He can get a sweet out of its paper, one hand holding, the other unwrapping. He can wash and dry his hands. He can put his shoes and socks on.

At three he climbs the stairs, one foot on each step, but on coming down he still puts both feet on each tread, sometimes holding the banister. When he gets to the bottom, he will probably jump the last step. He can now stand on one foot, briefly. He can ride a tricycle. He gets dressed on his own, except for those difficult buttons, but do not expect him to put his shoe on the correct foot. He can copy a circle when you ask him to and show him how it is done.

The four-year-old goes up and down stairs like you. He will skip on one foot. He can go to the toilet on his own and dress himself completely – unless a button is very stiff and new.

At five he is well away. He ties his shoelaces, skips on either foot, draws a triangle with a pencil. From now on it is physical education, dancing, games – fun things, using and practising motor skills.

Unwanted movements: tics and twitchings

77 Besides the development of normal movements, parents may observe their child making unwanted, useless movements. About a fifth of all schoolchildren twitch at some time. They show 'tics', purposeless flickerings in muscle groups. The usual cause is a stress at school or at home. It is no good saying, 'For heaven's sake, do stop making that silly face' – the poor child would if he could, but he can't. He may be able to exercise some control for a short time, but it does not last. The real cure is to find the cause and to get rid of that. It may turn out that a specific learning disability is at the root of the problem or it may be a purely emotional disturbance.

There is a rare condition in which the muscular tics persist over a long time and are associated with verbal or vocal ones. Not only can the child be seen to twitch, but he makes funny noises as well and may even swear quite surprisingly. There will be complaints from school about his behaviour and quite likely a specific retardation in reading and spelling. This is called the 'Gilles de la Tourette syndrome' after the doctor who first described it. If your child matches up to this description, you must seek advice from your family doctor. There are treatments and ways to help, not least of which is the recognition by teachers and parents of the nature of the disturbance.

There are other types of uncontrollable movements with a variety of causes. Rheumatic fever, cerebral palsy and epilepsy [120] may manifest themselves in this way. If your child makes silly movements repeatedly, consult your doctor.

Nelson was born by Caesarian section because the afterbirth was blocking the neck of his mother's womb. He was kept in special care for two weeks after that, but passed his 'milestones' at normal times.

He got on fine at the infants school, but when he was seven it was thought that he was failing to learn to read by his teachers, who referred him to the educational psychologist. She remarked on his nervousness, noted that he made 'silly' noises, could not relax and was trembling during her examination. He made exaggerated gestures, waved his arms around a lot and sucked his little finger. She felt he fluctuated between 'playing baby' and being mature and assertive. His non-verbal reasoning was average and she found that he had the perceptual ability to enable him to read. On the verbal side he did less well and was less than low average when it came to verbal reasoning. His memory was poor. She felt that his thinking powers were underdeveloped and that his attention was bad. In class, he made no proper use of special help offered and he was constantly disruptive, talking loudly and irrelevantly, making odd noises, and fidgeting and twitching.

When seen in the clinic at the age of eight and a half, he

had limited concentration, poor comprehension of what he heard and a poor auditory memory. The speech therapist saw no twitchings. The doctor found nothing amiss on clinical examination and also saw no twitchings or tics.

On the other hand, the remedial teacher found that his reading was two years behind the level for his age and the occupational therapist who tested his handwriting and spelling found that he had a spelling age of five and a half – in fact he could not spell. Both these investigators reported a lot of unwanted movements. He tossed his head to the left, stuck his tongue out repeatedly without any suggestion of being cheeky, and rose up in his seat as though he were 'posting' in a saddle.

After extensive investigations to eliminate any physical cause for his tics, the paediatrician concluded that they were nervous in origin, and to some extent situational. This was why the non-threatening doctor and speech therapist saw nothing amiss, while the remedial teacher and occupational therapist probing his weakest classroom skills were treated to an outburst of twitchings.

The child psychiatrist organized a supportive programme for him at the day hospital as she felt that nothing could be achieved at school until his nervousness had been investigated and relieved.

Testing for motor development

78 To be of value, tests of motor or any other element of development must be standardized. That is, the test must have been given to a large number of children so that the performance which a normal child will achieve at a given age may be determined. It is no good thinking that most seven-year-olds can do this or that. What they can actually do must be found out by a properly conducted scientific survey of a large group.

There are three types of test which specialists use to estimate a child's motor development.

The first is a general test of total development: vision, speech, hearing, movement, toilet training, the lot. This sort of test always contains within it some sub-tests of the various aspects of motor development. It is the category of test which the doctor in the child welfare clinic does routinely when screening a baby's general health and progress.

The second is a test to investigate a specific problem, but it contains an element of motor activity. For example, the Frostig Test of Visual Perception requires among other things that the child should connect two widely spaced objects by drawing a line between two guidelines without touching either. As the test progresses, the guidelines become closer together. Inability to wield a pencil because of clumsiness lowers the score.

The third is a test of what the child can do using many aspects of motor development: balance, hand and leg coordination, finger movements, rhythms; movement and static control.

The disadvantages of any of these tests are many. A child's reaction to the artificial situation is a variable. So, too, is the child's past experience. Cultural activities may distort the results unless these have been taken into account during the standardization of the test. The impartiality of the tester should be without doubt, but everyone who carries out these tests is aware of possible observer error.

Comparing one test result with another several months later is a more reliable method of reaching a conclusion than taking one isolated reading.

The uses made of the test results vary with the training of the tester. Doctors see motor tests not only as indications of development but also as possible pointers towards diseases which may be present; their main interest lies in identification of physical abnormalities. Psychologists are aware that delays in motor development may be associated with behavioural disturbances and with low levels of intelligence. They may use the tests as part of a general assessment of a child's emotional development.

Physiotherapists and occupational therapists are concerned with treatment. Their use of tests is slanted towards determining suitable therapy programmes and also as checks of the success of their activities.

Do not forget that all professional testers rely heavily on the parents' view of the child, so do not hesitate to tell them what you have seen the child doing.

Right, left and crossed laterals

There are three different conditions which are related to learning disabilities. These are: the confusion between right and left; ambidexterity; and crossed laterals. It is important that parents understand what these words imply.

79

Right and left

Take the business of knowing right from left. By the age of four, a third of all children can say which is their right hand. By six, this number has doubled and quite a few can point to their right foot with their left hand when asked to do so. An eight-year-old should be able to distinguish right from left on himself and many can indicate which is which on someone else. The child who confuses right from left on himself after the age of eight has some degree of delay in development. It may be associated with difficulty in naming colours or a poor understanding of what 'in front', 'behind', 'under' and 'over' mean. (There is very rarely a problem with 'up' or 'down'.) In such cases, help is needed and a speech therapist is the person to consult. She can tell if there is a specific language delay. If she feels that it is the child's intelligence which is at fault, she may recommend that a psychologist be consulted to establish the IQ.

Ambidexterity

Knowing right from left is quite different from preferring to use your right hand rather than your left for skilled jobs. All children pass through a stage of being ambidextrous, or rather ambi-non-dextrous, before becoming definitely right- or left-handed. If you watch your three-month-old baby, you will see that he uses both his hands indiscriminately. By nine months, one hand leads when he reaches for a toy. The two-year-old should leave you in no doubt as to which is his dominant hand. Ninety per cent of us end up right-handed. A few children remain ambidextrous for some time. This is not an advantage. It suggests some degree of neurological immaturity.

Crossed laterals

If a child has a dominant eye on one side and a dominant hand or foot on the other, he is said to have mixed dominance, or crossed laterals. There is no anatomical difference between him and the child who is firmly right- or left-side dominant. There is a shift of preference rather than a change in the nerve fibres leading to and from the brain. There is a well-established belief that crossed laterals have a direct relation to learning disabilities: 'Have crossed laterals, be a poor reader or speller.' The odd thing is that only two thirds of right-handers are also right-eyed. This means that over twenty-five per cent of the population are right-handed and left-eyed. They have mixed dominance. Not all have learning disabilities.

Perhaps a very important factor is the role of the ears. We are all either right- or left-ear dominant. It is much more difficult to establish which ear is dominant than it is to identify the preferred hand or eye. An observer can ask a child to perform a number of motor tasks involving the use of one member only and from this judge where there is any crossed laterality. It is not easy to do this with hearing and the ears. But, as far as language and reading are concerned, the interest in ear laterality lies in the presence of language centres in one or other cerebral hemisphere [55, 56, 57] and the use made by the learning child of the different capabilities of those halves of the brain. It is possible that right-ear dominance promotes fast, inaccurate reading, linguistic skills being used at the expense of visuo-spatial ones, while left-ear dominance promotes slow, accurate reading with great attention being paid to the shape and form of the letters and words.

The problem is bedevilled by the brain's capability of switching dominant sides in the face of disease. This certainly applies to the eye and possibly to the ear as well.

From a practical point of view it is best to regard crossed laterality as an at-risk factor and check the child's physical condition in case there is an associated disease process – anything from mild brain damage to poor visual acuity.

All in all, crossed laterality is a topic which becomes more difficult to understand the more closely we grapple with it.

Helping with right/left confusion, ambidexterity and crossed laterals

There are plenty of ways in which physiotherapists, occupational therapists and physical education teachers can help to improve spatial awareness and promote laterality. It has to be done with care. Everyone has heard of the left-handed child, forced to be right-handed for social reasons, developing a stammer. While this is not inevitable, it is important not to impose unnecessary stress. The therapists aim, in their movement programmes, to increase the efficiency of the child's doing, to improve his own body awareness. They give him a sense of achievement and at the same time improve his language development by relating what they are saying to what he is doing.

80

They do not have a direct effect on his reading and spelling, because crossed laterals, ambidexterity and right/left confusion are not causes of learning disabilities but symptoms produced by what is sometimes a common cause.

Not all left-handed children are dyslexic and left handedness cannot be regarded as a cause of dyslexia. It is, however, often associated with handwriting problems, either because the child has not been taught appropriately or because he is clumsy as well. The capabilities of the left-handed child have to be carefully assessed to find out whether any other problems, for instance of language, are present as well.

The child should be equipped with left-handed tools, a pen and scissors being the most important. The telephone directory of any of the larger cities usually contains the address of a 'left-handed' shop where these may be bought.

A conscious effort on the part of the teacher and the parent must be made to show the child how to hold and use the pen [185, 186]. If they are really stuck, the occupational therapy department of the local hospital should be able to help out, but it may be necessary to be referred there by the family doctor.

Summary (76–80)

By the age of eight a child should know the difference between his own right and left.

By two it should be obvious whether a child is going to be right- or left-handed.

Right/left confusion, ambidexterity and crossed laterals are not causes of learning disabilities; they are associated symptoms.

Exercises help to improve body image, spatial relationships, language and self-esteem. They do not improve reading and spelling. Teaching does this.

Clumsiness

81 It is one thing to read a list of milestones before the birth of your baby or during that first fine flush of parenthood immediately after the happy event. It is quite another to recognize when your child is becoming 'clumsy'. Rarely is a milestone passed suddenly. A child's capabilities vary from day to day. Illness may hold things up. A spell in bed from a chesty cough may not have any specific effect but it will alter the pattern of development slightly.

The realization that their child is clumsy creeps up slowly on parents and it may not be until your child gets to school that his poor skills become obvious to everyone, including the child. A mother may unwittingly slow down a child's development by doing things for him. In the rush and bother of going somewhere ('Quick, your father's waiting'), it is easy to put on his shoes, tie the laces, speed the dressing process. Valuable practice time may be lost to the child and he may come to stand passively waiting for 'Mummy do it'. We are all clumsy at some stage; manual skills and coordination take time to develop. There is a gradient from skilfulness to clumsiness, and clumsiness takes many forms. A child may be generally uncoordinated. He may tumble a lot and be covered in bruises. He may have difficulty in learning to ride a bike, turn a somersault, walk along a low wall, be good enough at ball games to be included in teams. A child may have poor hand skills. Food goes all over the place and it is tempting to keep a bib on him longer than usual; if he can knock over his mug, he does. He cannot tie knots. He does not hold his pencil properly; he writes badly. Games played with a small ball, like table tennis, are a nightmare. He may excel at swimming or long-distance running.

The speech therapists recognize a particular form of tongue clumsiness; the child knows what he wants to say but it does not come out right. Articulation is poor. There may be an underlying neurological problem. Speech therapy often helps.

The clumsy child needs investigation because clumsiness has many different causes.

Causes of clumsiness

The causes of clumsiness may be divided into two groups; medical and not-so-medical.

82

A large number of physical diseases may result in a child being clumsy. These include localized brain damage, cerebral palsy, general conditions like St Vitus' dance associated with rheumatic fever, and inherited muscular weaknesses.

The not-so-medical conditions are more difficult to define, treat and recognize. They fall into two types.

There are some children who are clumsy but have no learning disabilities. Because a child is clumsy, he does not have to have classroom problems. The mathematical genius may not shine on the football field. Being an egghead has its compensations, though there may be some agonies at those times when physical prowess seems to be important.

There are some children who are clumsy and have learning disabilities but who do not have any specific medical condition. Why? It is known that clumsiness occurs more frequently among boys than girls; that children with low IQs are more likely to be clumsy than those with high ones; that children of low birth-weight are more likely to be clumsy than those of normal weight; that emotional factors play a big part. In the same sort of way that worry can give certain types of adults ulcers, so can tension, unhappiness and stress produce clumsiness in children. It would be easy if *all* the children with these factors were clumsy and did badly when trying to learn to read and spell. But this is not so. There is an association between those conditions and clumsiness and learning disabilities, but no more than that. So what causes clumsiness? There are times when the specialists chicken out of being definite because they do not have sufficient proof to be anything other than vague. This is one of those times. Clumsiness with learning difficulties but no obvious physical disease may be the result of very mild brain damage that hardly shows; it may be something which runs in the family or is inherited in the genetic make-up of the child; it may be a combination of these last two together with a low I Q; it may be something to do with being a boy and not a girl. Altogether, this is an unsatisfactory state of knowledge, or rather of ignorance.

Parental action regarding clumsiness

83 It may be that, during the course of the routine health screening of your child, the doctor at the baby or child development clinic sees that there may be some delay in motor development. But if you have noticed clumsiness, he may refuse to perform in the doctor's office, in the consulting room, or he may put on an extra good performance, almost to your chagrin. Do not omit to tell the doctor of your worries and what you have seen. The doctor needs to know what your child is like every day. If, however, clumsiness becomes apparent to you, probably underlined by the remarks made by grannies, play-group leaders or class teachers, then get your child checked out medically. Do not wait, hoping that it will all get better on its own. If the doctor thinks that there may be an underlying physical cause he will investigate matters further for you. Do not be ashamed to bring the child back a second time if nothing definite is found at first. Delays in development become apparent as time passes, and the comparison between the findings at one examination with those at another after an interval of time may be much more revealing than an isolated check-up. The treatment depends on the cause.

Helping clumsy children

84 If there is a medical cause for the clumsiness, treatment must be in the hands of the doctor, physiotherapist and occupational therapist. This team will devise an appropriate programme of help, both for specific parts of the body and also for the overall skills and dexterity of the child. They will be prepared to give you and the class teacher advice, so that the particular disability can be dealt with and its effects in the home and classroom minimized. If there is no truly medical cause for the clumsiness, the two therapists will still be of value. Not only will their training programmes increase the child's awareness of the environment and develop his motor skills, but their wide use of language and the sense of achievement which they instil in the child will increase his overall abilities. Parents are eager to contribute what they can, either by doing things with the child or by paying for extra help, perhaps dancing class, eurythmy, judo or swimming. Super. There are two warnings to heed.

First, if you want to do something with your clumsy child to improve his dexterity, be sure to pick a subject which interests him and which he is good at. Children need to practise acquired skills as well as learn new ones, so let him show off to you. Fun must predominate; forget the business of teaching him anything at home. It is with you that practice will make perfect. Leave it to the professionals to introduce new skills.

Secondly, if you are going to arrange other activities for him, make sure that he has individual help first before he goes into a group. Coming up against a lot of well-coordinated children will do nothing for his self-confidence, and if he has any sense he will just go on strike and refuse to make a fool of himself in front of his mates. There is a lot which can be done to help, but remember, no one ever learnt to spell by jumping up and down on a trampoline; the hard graft has still to be done.

Summary (81–4)
There are many different reasons why a child may be clumsy.
Clumsiness by itself does not cause dyslexia.
Clumsiness and dyslexia may be caused by the same condition.
If your child is clumsy, get a doctor to check him out.
Exercise programmes may help clumsiness but will have only an indirect benefit for the dyslexic child.

Chapter Nine
Language

Introduction

Language is the expression of thought and feeling. It is a system of symbols and signs, with rules for communication. It is a process aimed at conveying meaning. Any message is based on the meaning of the words or gestures used and is dependent on the experience of both the sender and the receiver.

There are three main forms of language: spoken, written and body language. Only the first two use words.

An adult receives language through his ears, eyes and, if blind, fingers. He takes the message to pieces and decodes it. Then he responds, using the same language to express his meaning.

The child must learn to do this. He needs the right sort of model from which to acquire experience of language. He needs to have intact mechanisms for receiving, decoding, encoding and expressing.

In the context of this book we have dealt mainly with the development of language in the child and what affects it, for good or ill.

Language in the adult

85 We both listen and read in order to extract meaning from the continuum of speech or print. If we have some idea of what the message is likely to be and the form it will take (after all, the language heard in church is different from that of the supermarket) we can more readily understand it. Anticipation of language patterns (which are determined by situation and language rules) will help us predict what words will come next. As the message proceeds, each word or syllable is successfully understood. This success allows the listener, or reader, to predict accurately the next larger group of words. The larger group of words in turn narrows down the range of possible choices as to what the total message might be.

A crude analogy can be made with going for a long drive. At first the driver seeks the M-way signs saying 'The North/The West'; a little later names of cities are picked out; near the exit point names of small towns are focused on; finally in the village the particular house name is found.

In short, the hearer or reader with an intact and sophisticated language system will make use of the broad pattern of the words heard or written in the sentence to help him decode the smaller components, such as words, syllables and even phonemes (the distinct units of sound: there are about forty in English). This will be done in preference to starting from the detailed small constituents of the message and building up the whole. Various items of information have to be held in the memory as they are progressively processed and re-processed. But the capacity of short-term memory [73] seems limited at best to nine items. Therefore items have to be amalgamated into larger coherent units, as necessary. In practice, smaller units are amalgamated not only into larger units but also more meaningful ones. Consequently single sounds or letters are grouped into meaningful parts of words (for example, prefixes like dis- or pre-, suffixes like -ed or -ing), then into complete words, then into sentences.

The skills involved in processing receptive language, both oral and silent (listening and reading), are closely interrelated with considerable overlap between them, and are not to be separated from expressive language, both oral and silent (speaking and writing).

Reading is understanding visually, as distinct from auditorily, signalled language; it amounts to thinking under the stimulus of print. It is closely connected with talking, especially in the early stages. Expressive language has several aspects: the semantic (meaning), the grammatical/syntactic (how to organize words into meaningful messages), the phonological (noises) and articulatory (how to make the noises), and spelling and handwriting.

As has been said earlier, the receptive and expressive aspects of language are inseparable, like the two halves of a dual carriageway. Remember the cycle tracks along each side? They are for non-verbal communication: facial expression, body posture, gesture, mime, intonation and rhythm, and drawing. Note that all these, bar one, are mediated through vision and movement. The auditory exception, intonation and rhythm, must be learnt and used in the appropriate way if the loosely structured sequence of phrases and clauses that make up spoken language is to be understood. Drawing, if figurative, connects directly with the semantic aspects of oral and silent language.

The model

The child's mother must provide the warm, comfortable model from whom the child learns and who gives him a complete sense of security **86** and dependence. Without her presence he has no model and no stimulus for the development of his own language. There are other, potentially hazardous, factors.

A very large family is in some sense a disadvantage for its individuals. Not only those older than the child, but also those coming after him, make demands on the mother and steal her attention from him. The maternal cake is only so big. An older sister may do her best, at least some of the time, but . . .

Physical or mental illness in the mother may affect her ability to communicate with her child. If she has a longstanding disability which has been obvious before the birth of her baby, then provision can be made to support them both. More difficult to cope with is the situation arising when the mother is suddenly and unexpectedly prevented from bonding with her baby. Nurses, however nice, are not a patch on mum – they go off duty; she never does. The attraction that a baby exerts for most of us is not the same as mother-love and is no substitute for it. Dramatic maternal illness after the birth is obvious and steps are taken to provide as good a surrogate as possible for the mother who suffers some obstetric disaster. But things may creep up surreptitiously. Puerperal depression comes into this category and is of the greatest importance as it will hold up the infant's development of language. For hormonic reasons beyond the mother's control, she may become so depressed and miserable during the first few weeks of her baby's life that she is unable to do more than change the nappy and push the bottle at him. Not only complete misery but a total inability to think and to organize herself may paralyse her. Things can get so bad that she wants to kill herself or the baby. Psychiatric help will rescue both of them. While it is becoming effective for her, a surrogate mum must be arranged for him. A break in the chain of events which foster language and emotional development can take a surprisingly long time to repair.

Emotional stress within the family may reflect on all its members, none more than the developing child. The solution of separation and divorce, though relieving the parents of intolerable tensions, may produce such anxiety in a child that development of learning may be delayed [127]. The result is a learning disorder of environmental origin, in contrast with a learning disability of biological origin.

Mother tongue versus school tongue

87 When both parents speak a language other than that spoken at school, their child will obviously have difficulty in class. If he has cracked the code of his mother tongue, then he will have a model on which to build the outside, or foreign, language, like putting scaffolding round an extant building. He will overcome his early difficulties if given proper teaching. The degree to which he overcomes them will of course vary from one child to the next, but on the whole in Great Britain children whose mother tongue is not English do better in public examinations, for subjects which are not language-based, that is, mathematics and related subjects rather than English or history. This does not prevent them from doing well in examinations for their own language, particularly if they have been attending classes in their mother tongue and related culture. A number of ethnic minorities run Saturday or after-school classes of this kind, generally with great success.

Children whose mother's *own* mother tongue is English do better than children whose mother is using English as her second language. It is hard to croon to your baby in a foreign language, difficult to sing nursery rhymes to him in any other way than your mother sang to you. It is well-nigh impossible to speak spontaneously in a foreign tongue so that not a trace of your own nursery language remains. Even when the mother speaks English spontaneously, she may not use the same English as her child will encounter at school. The sounds of her speech, the stresses on various parts of words, the actual words and the way she puts words together to make sentences may all be different from those of the teacher. So at first the child finds the teacher difficult to understand, though he does not realize this.

When Sandy came to the clinic a short time ago he was said to have 'a word-finding problem perhaps of significance', the 'perhaps' indicating that he had a delay in the development of language. The standardized test used elsewhere to determine his level of language development had required him to choose one of four pictures which showed a scarecrow, and he had been unable to do so. There are, of course, precious few scarecrows north of the Scottish–English border, and when asked to point at the picture of a 'tattie-bogle' he got it in one. 'Yon teacher's a daftie, does she no ken a tattie-bogle?' The local education authority had, eventually, channelled him to a special class for children with important difficulties in auditory perception and language expression, for in South London his rich Glaswegian accent was as incomprehensible to teachers as to the other children.

Arguably a child with such an obvious and basic problem,

however it is labelled, will always be picked out and helped by the education authority. But a milder form of the same difficulty can be exacerbated by family expectation.

Mustafa was the younger son of a professional family who had settled in England before his birth. The language spoken in the home – and written, for it had a distinctive script – originated on the Indian subcontinent. His mother went back to work when Mustafa was four, leaving him with an English-speaking childminder. At five he started school in English. He was a dear little boy, cheerful, friendly and communicative, who often did not understand a question or instructions for a task. His conversation consisted of fragmentary phrases, grammatically incorrect, backed up by many delightful smiles. Although his oral reading of stories was a trifle better than average for both accuracy and comprehension of what he read, his spelling was very poor. Investigation showed that he had a very immature grasp of English sound–symbol association and had no idea what a rhyme was (a most necessary prop to spelling in the early stages); weakest of all was his understanding of English words [90]. No wonder his teachers complained that this seemingly very bright little boy (an informal assessment supported this impression) was constantly getting hold of the wrong end of the stick and that his reading progress had stopped, having apparently reached a plateau.

No matter, you might say, he is young, and a bit ahead of average. But his anxious parents expected him to streak ahead, on the way to an eventual professional qualification to be obtained in England. It was suggested that he needed a lot more informal English, best obtained by spending the long summer holidays speaking English with native English speakers. His mother demurred: all the family's social contacts were with other immigrants. What about a junior school teacher to play with him for a few hours each day? This suggestion was acceptable to the family.

The child and language

88 A child must be able to hear and see normally if the messages from the outside world are to reach his brain in normal form, have a normal effect and stimulate normal language development. Disease may alter the contribution from the ears and eyes, affect the brain and have an impact on development before and after birth, and on functioning in childhood.

Diseases affecting the brain may distort the ways in which incoming messages can be dealt with. The decoding process may be affected and comprehension thereby limited. The child's ability to say what he wants to, so that everyone else can understand, may be limited. There may be difficulty in making the tongue or limbs work as desired, difficulty in perceiving shapes and letter formations, or subtle weaknesses such as an inability to find the right word at the right moment. Some brain malfunctions are obvious at birth; others only become apparent when reading, writing or spelling are attempted. Simultaneously the child has to learn and use non-verbal language. To acquire these interconnected skills the child must be intact.

In the authors' opinion a child is not born with a sophisticated language system. To acquire it he must have, for oral language, auditory perception, discrimination, synthesis, sequencing and memory, and analogous visual mechanisms for written language. Adequate acuity, both auditory and visual, is dependent on the structure of speech and vision organs being normal and the neuro-motor system being correctly coordinated.

In developmental terms, the steps a child goes through to acquire verbal language follow a well-signposted hierarchical path: to begin with, the child must hear what people are saying, that is, he must take in oral language. When his oral receptive language is on the way to being in good working order and he can accept and decode the message, he must, through understanding, return the message in the same code; he is then using oral expressive language.

So far he has dealt with the noisy language in the air and his hearing and noise-making anatomy have been put into practice. At the next, formally taught, stage, that of reading, he enters the realm of silent language, decoded through the eyes, but dependent for meaning on the experience he has had of oral, heard language. Writing, encoded in spelling, is silent expressive language. As the child develops language normally he becomes more adept at amalgamating, classifying and remembering what started as indistinct and separate language stimuli.

Summary (85–8)
An adult's language is his central communicative ability, consisting of spoken, written and body language.

An adult's language has grown out of his experience; he uses language to consolidate, clarify, enhance and anticipate experience.

A child must learn to communicate. To do so he needs to have intact mechanisms for receiving, decoding, analysing and expressing language.

A child must have the right model from whom to learn language.

A child needs appropriate experiences to stimulate language.

A mother tongue at variance with the language of instruction can be, but is not always, an educational handicap.

The parental contribution to a child's language development is crucial. It is the make-or-mar factor in their child's intellectual development.

Parents and their child's language

89 Detailed analysis of any child's language is a job for the speech therapists. Parents may read books on child development and find out how many words their young should be using and at what age, or when he should be making sentences. Such books are easy to read but difficult to put into practice. It helps to consider articulation and the noises a child makes. It is easier to gauge his output than it is to find out whether or not he understands what you are talking about. So we have not detailed his expected rate of vocabulary development – so much depends on the language used by parents, where you live and what is going on around you. The vocabulary of a farmer's son will be different from that used by the son of a capstan lathe setter. There is a section on how your child makes noises, one on the noises themselves, and then one on syntax in relation to the younger child. (Syntax is the organization of words in speaking and writing to make the message unambiguous.) Finally there is something about the child at school. This includes his use of 'proper' language, and the older child's silent language, both receptive and expressive.

The intention is to give parents some indication of what to expect and of danger signs which should alert them to a developing problem.

Vocabulary

90 The extent of a child's receptive vocabulary, that is, the words that he understands, and in large measure the concepts behind them, can be formally assessed [99] and a figure obtained. But a bald number, referring to single words known, is of limited use, because words are not often used – except by very young children – in isolation. They come in the context of a sentence or a phrase and at first understanding is approximate, gradually refining with repeated use. Words also come in the context of a situation, with the referent – the object or the experience – readily identifiable.

Think of a six-year-old taken for a camping holiday. At the end of it he will know the words for every specialized piece of equipment he has come across and he will discourse to admiring grandparents on their uses, respective merits and probably cost too. At home, if a child from the age of three upwards joins in cooking or gardening there are considerable opportunities for learning words with very specific meanings, such as 'egg-whisk', 'crumbly', 'trowel', 'pruning'.

The order in which children learn words from various categories varies. Observations, supported by research, suggests that words for movements are easy and therefore learnt early (though words for position come a little later), then words for shape, size or sound, then those for taste and texture (hence the use of cooking), then names for particular objects the child has used ('the naming of parts' is as necessary for children as for soldiers) or particular activities he has taken part in, for instance shelling peas.

In general, three factors will extend vocabulary: (a) the width of a child's experience; (b) the quality and amount of running commentary that goes with it; and (c) discussion of the same experience and subsequent reminders of it in conversation.

Commentary, discussion and reminiscence are means of thinking with other people, enabling the speaker to share his intuitive, implicit understanding of a situation; speech will make this understanding explicit to himself. A wide command of words will make the understanding sharper.

This does not mean that when a word or phrase has been used once or twice it will be permanently and correctly remembered, even if not actively used. Some words will be forgotten, rediscovered, re-learnt; gradually secondary and figurative meanings will be welded on to the first, with its obvious referent – think of 'puppet'. Spoken language (by which is meant vocabulary, syntax, intonation and articulation) within the home will always be what principally determines the child's breadth and use of vocabulary.

A difficulty in finding the right word to use may also be associated with

Low I Q [67]
English as a second language [87]
Occasionally some forms of brain damage [64]
Anxiety [128]

Katie's parents travelled some considerable distance to bring her to the clinic. They were exceedingly worried. Their only child, their darling little girl aged seven and very pretty, was not progressing with reading and had in the last twelve months become cross, miserable and uncooperative, alternating between noisy misery and puzzled withdrawal. Until then she had been so sweet, so biddable, so amusing. Amusing? Yes, when she started talking she called everything 'door', and playfully parents and grandparents had tagged along and 'doored' everything too. For how long? Oh, just about until she had started school.

On examination her language was found to be exceptionally immature, with a vocabulary barely equivalent to that of a three-year-old. We reckoned she was a remarkably good-natured child to have put up with so much school before becoming miserable and mutinous. Immediate speech therapy was prescribed.

The above is of course an extreme situation but one which could easily have been avoided.

Wendy was a pleasant little girl of seven, giggly and chatty, who lived in a prosperous suburb. Her school, well-known for its high achievements, had suggested that she should come to the clinic because her reading had stopped progressing and her spelling had never really got off the ground. Far too often she still spelt at random.

Her medical history revealed that she suffered from enlarged tonsils and adenoids, and (badly) from hay fever; for the last she took a decongestant, but this did nothing to improve her hearing. Her mother said that Wendy had never spoken in single words but had, at the age of two and a half, gone from silence straight into phrases.

Tests done at the clinic revealed that her auditory memory [73] was way behind what it should have been at her age and her attempts at auditory discrimination [99] were random guesswork rather than considered responses to clearly received stimuli. Her receptive vocabulary [103] was also a long way short of what would be expected. When she read a story and came to an unfamiliar word she would point to it and ask: 'What's that say?' Faced with a list of phonically regular words ('plod', 'dust') she would sound out the individual letters but was rarely able to put the letter sounds together into a word that she recognized. She could not recognize a rhyme or categorize any words by their sound.

Medical advice apart, her school was advised to encourage her to work on the meaning of words. The obvious strategy was, when reading continuous prose, to read to the end of the sentence and then work out the unfamiliar word first from the local context of the sentence and, if necessary, from the context of the whole story. The sound of the first letter of the word would act as a clue. For spelling it was suggested that she should tackle words with the same letter string, for example, 'angel', 'strange', 'arrange', 'danger', in order to get away from single-letter sounds and give her ear and eye a larger unit to work on. For the weekly 'spellings' she should be given a list of such words and their definitions, and the spelling tested by giving her the definition only and asking her to write the word.

Here was a child whose school had bandied about the word 'dyslexic' in relation to her poor spelling and halt in reading progress. Backtracking from this provisional diagnosis had revealed (a) an inability to segment and organize syllables; and (b) a significant shortfall in vocabulary.

Going one level further back, the medical information included a history of frequent bouts of hearing loss, due to middle-ear infection [31] and hay fever.

While poor vocabulary had put a kibosh on progress with reading (one kind of 'dyslexia'), the medical cause of the poor vocabulary had produced an additional form of 'dyslexia': random spelling.

Articulation

If you stand at the entrance to a cave and shout loudly, the echo of the words will bounce back to you clearly but the quality of your voice will be changed by the resonance of the cave. If the size and shape of the cave is altered by a rockfall or flooding, then the quality of the echo will change too.

When we speak, we are making noises at the entrance to our own private cave, formed by the nose and mouth. We can change its size and

91

shape by moving the lips, cheeks and tongue or by raising or lowering the jaw and soft palate. The soft palate lies right at the back of the roof of the mouth.

These mouth movements – articulation – alter the pattern of noise which comes up from the voice box. This Adam's apple or larynx lies in the neck. It determines the individual pitch of the voice, higher for girls than for boys. Articulatory movements alter the resonance of our cave and produce the different sounds of speech.

A child learns the right movements to make with his mouth and throat from the people around him, in particular his mother. He learns not only by listening but also by watching the muscle changes of her mouth and neck. His noises mimic hers. If her articulation is faulty, so will his be. If her voice is flat from depression or partial deafness, so will his be. If she does not talk to him much, he will be slow to learn to talk. To change from the reflex noises – like sucking and burping – to speech, the child's mouth and jaws must develop normally and his teeth must be in good shape.

Several things may affect the development of correct articulation:

1. malformation of parts of the mouth, hair lip, cleft palate, jaw deformities;
2. poor nerve control of mouth muscles due to paralysis, for example after an operation to the back of the throat;
3. brain damage affecting the pathways of instruction to the mouth muscles, so that correct instructions do not reach the mouth muscles;
4. damage to the mechanisms of sound reception or perception either at the ear or in the brain;
5. a faulty sound environment.

It is the specialist's and speech therapist's job to sort out what is wrong and why. Early treatment may work wonders. The later things are left, the harder it is to improve them.

Parents need some simple guidelines to tell them when they should be seeking advice:

- A two-year-old who only uses a few simple words singly, or who does not speak at all, must be investigated.
- A three-year-old who is not talking in sentences or whom the family finds difficult to understand must be investigated.
- A four-and-a-half-year-old whose speech is unintelligible to people not in his immediate family (including visiting grannies), or who stutters, must be investigated.

Articulation and spelling

Treatment has shown that training in auditory discrimination improves feedback and as a result leads to improvement in the articulation of single words, though it may not hold good for longer utterances.

92

Correct articulation has two pay-offs: (a) the speaker is intelligible to his audience; and (b) he will find correct spelling easier.

The five-year-old should be able to pronounce, for instance, 'slept' so that its five constituent sounds can be distinguished. At six or seven, he is more likely to write 'slept' with five letters, each with its distinct phonic value.

This becomes more important if the child attends a multinational school, like so many in our inner cities, where a simplified, pared-down form of English is the lingua franca of the playground. Words are ellided ('ordinary' is invariably 'ornery'), and endings showing the plurals of nouns; forms of verbs or adjectives; the distinction between adjective and adverb – all are lost. No matter, you may say, they still understand one another. So they do, but the language of instruction, of textbooks and audio-visual programmes is received English, precise and correct. The inaccurate or sloppy speaker often misses out on the finer shades of meaning carried by word endings. He is less likely to make use of the grammatical system of spelling [172]. Also, polysyllabic words will be a lot harder to segment into syllables ready for correct spelling. But regional accents are no bar to clear articulation; some, like that characteristic of Edinburgh, are of direct help in identifying consonants and so become a positive step towards spelling proficiency.

Gary was thirteen, large, cheerful and quite unworried about himself (except that he might possibly be overweight) and he reckoned he could always join his uncle in the latter's building business. His school and parents took a different view. He seemed bright enough, but was held back by his spelling. He'd had a lot of help with it in school, but it remained stubbornly imprecise. And yet his visual sequential memory [102] turned out to be fine and his handwriting very good. There were no complaints about his hearing, either.

He chattered readily but was hard to understand: he elided his words so that they ran into each other, consonant blends and clusters came out as one, the letter 't' was always glottal-stopped and all vowels came out as 'er'. During the spelling tests, he asked disarmingly for extra help: 'Did you say *regain* or *regained*?' – and he was quite able to sound the two distinctly.

It turned out that his spelling miscues were entirely due to inadequate auditory monitoring – unsurprising in view of his imprecise speech. We reminded him of 'The rain in Spain'. He was unimpressed.

93

Noises (speech sounds and their discrimination)

Not only does a child develop a vocabulary as he gets older, but he has to learn to cope with the noises which make up words. The ability to do this comes slowly, in fits and starts, and the range of what is a normal rate of progress is wide.

During the first eighteen months the average child acquires about fifty words, but they are not the same fifty words for all children. Each child is highly selective. The general sound pattern, however, is much the same with all children: 'a' as in 'mama' is the first vowel, followed by 'ee' as in 'feet' or 'oo' as in 'do'; 't' and 'k' are followed by 'h' and 'w'. There is a tendency to double up groups of sound: 'mam mama'. This initial development corresponds with the period of brain cell growth after birth and to the child's functional development.

After eighteen months there is a sudden jump in the size of his vocabulary; the child begins to use two words together as mini-sentences and there is an increase in his ability to distinguish between more closely similar noises. This goes on at the same time as he begins to label things. He gets better and better at this differentiation and the whole process may continue until he is three.

It is not possible to reproduce a sound accurately if it has not been clearly heard in the first place. 'Perception facilitates production', not the other way about. 'Listen Johnny, not wag – bag' as an approach does not work until Johnny knows the difference between 'w' and 'b', and that only happens when his brain cells have matured enough to enable him to do so.

Because each child is a selective listener, personal habits abound in the early years, depending on what he has been listening to.

It is easier for parents to recognize what their child is saying than to find out which noises he can hear and to differentiate between. So it is worth having a rough idea of what you should hear from him.

By three, all the vowel sounds should have been mastered (they are always present before the consonants); nasal sounds like 'm', 'n' and 'ng' in 'thing' should have followed; 'p', 't' and 'k' are acquired early. However, local dialects may have a delaying effect for some noises. By four, many blends of sound can be heard, so that the 'pl' of 'plod' and the 'st' of 'stop' are obvious. After four the 'sl' in 'slow' and the 'sw' in 'swing' are acquired. 'Ch', 'th' and 'j' come later.

Even so, these are general rules. The acquisition of different sounds creeps on slowly and there are many individual variations. Nursery rhymes said by mum and repeated by the child are a great help. 'Ride *a* cock horse to Banbury Cross' deals with a nice lot of vowel sounds. If it is blends you are after, try:

> Old mother Shuttle
> Lived in a coal-scuttle
> Along with her dog and her cat.
> What they ate I can't tell
> But 'tis known very well
> That none of the party was fat.

This sort of development goes on until the child is about seven or eight, when he should be able to produce all the sounds of English, with his appropriate regional variations. For example, in the south-east of England confusion between 'v', 'th' and 'f' goes on well into adult life, while in some parts of Scotland vowels are vastly preferred to consonants – 'oo' equals 'wool'. Difficult words to pronounce are difficult for all of us, especially children, so errors do occur. Between six and twelve the ability to put stresses in just the right place develops, and by the time logical thought is taking place the sounds of the language should have been mastered.

Something about syntax

Syntax is the correct construction of sentences, the right style to use when speaking or writing. It is the organization of language and so embodies a set of rules for a language. A child develops a grasp of syntax slowly and by stages. The bounds of normality are wide and there is no neat cut-off point when one stage or other will be reached. Listening to a child developing language is like looking at a river from the air: there are fast runs, wide slow-moving stretches, eddies, currents, twists and turns, but a general direction towards the sea. Some knowledge of the various stages helps a parent to identify delays in language development and will be useful to those who have no older child to serve as a model.

From birth to eighteen months, the child begins to use single

94

words, but each with a wealth of possible meaning. Each word may be a sentence in itself, interpretation being left to the adult listener. This may be difficult for strangers because a child may label something with a 'wrong' word, perhaps a verb for a noun, easily understood by the family but a puzzle to everyone else. These single words are used as commands, demands, greetings and, less often, as questions.

By two years old, two words are put together as observations when the child sees something: 'Dada gone'; or as questions: 'Where Mummy?'; or as a demand: 'Me down'. 'In' and 'on' are the first prepositions produced during this phase.

During the next six months, three words will be put together, so that recognizable sentences appear: 'Where that pussy?'; 'Put dolly bed'; 'Sit on Daddy'. Questions, demands and comments become more clearly differentiated. Blending of already used words continues and an increasing knowledge of words expands the range, especially when it comes to saying what he does not want to do: 'Me not want to'. By the age of three, statements, questions and commands are clearly expounded.

After three, the child learns the connecting words which join two or more simple sentences: 'Pussy eating 'cos she's hungry.' The word of the moment is 'and'. It appears all the time and keeps the child talking in the centre of the stage. Fiction follows fact, both joined by 'and'. It does not matter much as long as your child is talking and you are listening, and it's all for the fun of it.

The child of three and a half makes lots of mistakes. Pronouns get gorgeously abused. 'This' and 'that' mean much the same thing. The right order of adjectives is established: 'my big blue ball' not 'my blue big ball'.

About a year later 'I are' should be replaced by 'I am', past tenses are used properly and it is difficult to spot grammatical errors. What is still lacking is the ability to string sentences together to get over a full message.

Between the age of five and puberty, more and more ways of connecting sentences are used. Adverbs become familiar tools. Changing the stress of a sentence by altering the word order, perfection in the use of irregular words, comprehension of adult phrases formerly used parrot fashion – all these take place over six or seven years and are influenced by what is heard and what is read.

Teenagers will also learn the more subtle conventions of oral language: how interpolations ('comment clauses') like 'I mean', 'you see', 'mind you', 'tell me', can, by their position, refine the emphasis of the main sentence; how the comment clauses are signs that the speaker is relaxing, giving the listener time to catch up on the meaning. The speaker may also use 'fillers', like 'sort of', or repeat in different words what he has said earlier. These ploys give the speaker and the listener time to think, without drawing attention to the interval being given to thought. A pause at the beginning of the sentence suggests that the speaker is thinking how to express one idea in a sentence; a pause somewhere in the sentence suggests he is seeking *le mot juste*. A pause for dramatic effect again depends on its placing for the impression produced.

Written language in junior school

95 It starts with writing one's name. JIM in shaky capitals can be a form of self-assertion, or it may mean 'Remember Jim', or 'Don't touch Jim's bricks.' One-word written messages, like one-word utterances, need interpretation. The progression is to more explicit messages, like 'Love Jim.' Once he starts school there will be labelling. Cut-out pictures need naming: car – house – duck – tree. He will draw his own pictures, tell the teacher what they're about, she will write the caption and he will copy it below: 'My new bike'. From this it is an easy step to the diary, 'making personal statements' as the jargon has it, like: 'We had a bonfire, fireworks and sausages', and with luck he will be able to write 'we', 'had', 'a', 'and' from memory. Diary entries gradually become longer, almost imperceptibly; sometimes, with the aid of sequences of pictures, they turn into stories. Increased experience of stories, hearing them and telling his own, make the child's command of story-writing that much surer. Spelling and handwriting can be powerful stumbling blocks, but microcomputers ease the first and eliminate the second. Topic work brings in expository prose, which in junior school covers recording of observation and re-telling of facts in his own words.

Language in secondary school

96 Transfer to secondary school may give the child his first taste of close teacher control of discussion. This he sometimes translates into stilted written language: he stays with well-practised phrases and constructions and self-corrects for details. As he comes to feel more confident in his new surroundings he takes the risk of expressing strongly held views. On the basis of these and his own immediate experience, he writes enthusiastically. This is often very successful as long as he avoids imitation of what he thinks are more advanced forms of expression.

With time his own efforts (not least with writing) make him more dextrous with words; he will encompass detailed, precise observation with freshness of expression and start developing his own independent writing style. His confidence may stretch to humorous writing, perhaps re-telling amusing anecdotes. Getting these down on paper is often a collaborative task, interlaced with much discussion. In general, conversations should become more reflective, since widening interest in relationships beyond school and home leads to more comparing, contrasting, synthesizing. This enables him to look at his own experience from various angles; it also brings awareness and imitation of various fictional methods, depending on the audience being addressed.

The next stage is more reflective still. An important development is the growing child's ability to detach himself from a given subject. Consequently in writing, the expression of enthusiasm (which earlier may have lacked coherence) is now controlled for structure and detail. This raised level of accomplishment in expressing what he stoutly feels or believes will enhance his sense of his own personality. In reading, he is expected to 'interrogate the text' independently: to identify the clues to the most important symbols in the text, the purposes of the writer, to examine the values reflected. Two conversational demands arise: the first is greater awareness of his audience; the second is 'thinking on his feet', which amounts to being much quicker and more pertinent in developing an argument by referring to and extending what has been said earlier.

Before the start of university, conversational competence stretches to entering easily into other people's experiences or point of view, and perhaps revising his own; he shares ideas; he shifts readily from abstract concept to imaginative interpretation of personal knowledge; he builds complex arguments. He is a shrewd reader: he can read between and beyond the lines and so size up a writer's motives, aims and point of view. When writing, his factual reports are objective, impersonal, economically worded and unmistakably clear. On a topic he feels strongly about, his commitment, however vehement, is expressed with precision and subtlety. Depending on purpose he side-steps between styles: the transactional, the narrative, the personal, even the poetic.

In his adult life he will continue to demonstrate the inextricable links between listening, talking, reading and writing, as he melds them into mastery of communication. This is the tool with which the individual, from childhood, builds up his own intellectual and moral abilities. The potential for parental contribution is enormous.

Summary (86–96)

A child learns to talk from his mother.

If she has to be absent for some time, someone else who cares must take her place.

An ounce of mum at the start is worth a ton of speech therapy or remedial teaching later.

A child learns the sounds of speech from the noises his mother makes.

To do this he must be able to hear properly.

He learns to speak by copying his mother.

If he speaks badly, he should see the speech therapist.

By the age of five he should be able to make good sentences.

After five, his sentences should get longer and more complicated.

By the age of eight, he should be able to make all the sounds of English.

The more he reads, the better his spoken English will become.

Making correct speech sounds helps to make good spelling.

Is he slow with talking?

97

A mother may fear that her child is behind with his language development, seeing that he is not as advanced as the other children in the neighbourhood or in the play-group. She may have older ones with whom to compare him and recognize that he is not as far advanced as they were at the same age. If inappropriate help is sought, soothing reassurances may be made: 'It is because his sisters do all the talking for him'; 'He always gets what he wants without talking, he understands what we say'; 'He is the silent one of the family, just like his Uncle Arthur.'

A child with language delay may reach infant school at five without any adult having felt that it was worth doing anything to help. It will take the teacher a little while to become familiar with him and to suspect that there may be a problem. She may feel that the delay she sees is only temporary and that with a bit of individual help the child will catch up. If there is doubt, the speech therapist must be consulted.

In the United Kingdom it is perhaps unfortunate – anyway from the child's point of view – that the speech therapist is employed by the local health authority, while the educational psychologist works for the local education authority. This means that teachers are more likely to turn to the psychologist for help and advice, when the problem may lie in a different but complementary field and they would be better advised to consult a speech therapist.

The speech therapist

98 Put out of your mind the old-fashioned idea that the speech therapist is there to cure stammering and stuttering. Though she may help with such problems, her main interest is in the child's development of language. She brings to bear her specific expertise and training in the field, something which doctors, teachers and psychologists do not possess though all three disciplines have more than a nodding acquaintance with it. Her opinion on that subject necessarily overrides that of the others. She will identify precisely where the problem lies, and then either take the child on for therapy herself, or advise parents and teachers how best to proceed at home and in the classroom.

The speech therapist investigates verbal communication. A number of processes are involved, and their interaction can be described as a double chain joined into a circle. Consider first the circle. It is necessary to have experienced verbal communication over a period and to be able to hear it before it can be understood. After understanding what is heard, some idea or concept has to be made and related to other, already accepted, information. This is followed by the response, the desire to express oneself through articulation at the right moment (it's no use talking to thin air). This opportunity leads back to the experience of verbal language.

Now think of the two chains making up the circle. There is first an automatic level of verbal functioning, where heard and seen information has to be dealt with in the right order; the second chain corresponds to the meaningful level, where incoming and outgoing material has to be decoded and encoded, using the same code as that of the audience, in order to transmit ideas and thoughts.

With such a complicated set of processes to be investigated, the speech therapist prefers to do it 'properly', in depth, if circumstances allow. It may take her several hours with the child to understand fully what has happened to his language. She will need time with him alone, talking to and with him, but she may wish to go into the classroom or the home to see how he copes in social situations. She may wish to record him. She will use standardized tests as a framework on which to hang her opinion, but her clinical judgement and know-how are of much greater importance and enable her to give considered advice. In this way she compares with the psychologist, whose report on a child is as important as the figures she obtains for his IQ [70]. Again, like the clinical psychologist, the speech therapist will have to decide whether the language immaturity or deviation is due to (a) a disability of biological or psychiatric origin, and therefore in need of medical intervention first; or (b) a disorder, due to some social, familial or scholastic circumstance, in which case the social and educational services will be called upon first.

In both cases a learning difficulty will have been the first symptom of the learning disability or disorder. Administratively, the speech therapist is able to make direct contact with the appropriate medical, educational or social services, as the particular case may require. As well as investigating a child's language development, she will also concern herself with his listening skills, his ability to accept the verbal barrage which adults fire at him; for if a child cannot cope with the flow of words, then he will not be able to understand what is being said to him [31, 73].

Tests used by speech therapists

The speech therapist has a considerable number of tests at her command. **99** These investigate particular areas of auditory functioning: there are several tests of auditory discrimination (the child hears pairs of words and has to say whether the words are the same or different); several tests for investigating particular areas of syntactical competence; tests for various types of auditory memory, for the ability to organize auditory stimuli, for blending of letter sounds, and for vocabulary. She will use these as she thinks necessary. Some of these tests are 'open', that is, they can be used by others who are not trained speech therapists [103].

The speech therapist will want to assess the child's expressive ability. She will carry materials to get him talking: toys, single pictures (funny pictures of the 'what's wrong?' type are very good for obtaining an illuminating sample of verbal response); a series of pictures that first have to be put in sequence and then the story told, as in the comparable sub-test of the W I S C-R test [69], with perhaps an extra surprise picture offering an alternative conclusion; a story sequence of pictures presented one at a time with repeated sets of questions seeking particular responses (interpreting the picture, predicting the next, etc.).

Speech therapists also use Language Acquisition Remediation Speech Programme (L A R S P), devised by David Crystal. This makes a very detailed analysis of everyday speech, including 'ums', 'ers', repetitions and mistakes. The analysis reveals whether language development is retarded or deviant, and in precisely what respects. A remediation programme can then be based on the analysis. Obviously, L A R S P is a most time-consuming procedure; in practice the degree of detail it provides is necessary only in cases of extreme difficulty with expressive speech.

A battery of screening tests

100 If pressed for time, the speech therapist will use a battery of screening tests: tests of speech sound discrimination, articulatory sequencing, grammatical closure, and so on. The two most commonly used ones are described below.

The Reynell

The Reynell Development Language Scales (revised) are suitable for testing children aged from one to six, but are at their most illuminating with children aged one to four. They are designed for use with children who are suspected of having some language deficit and consist of three sections:

1. Verbal comprehension, which has ten parts in increasing order of development, starting with the child's ability to recognize some word patterns, going on to the interpretation of different parts of speech and finally to the stage when the child uses language as a way of understanding what he and others are thinking.

2. Verbal comprehension again, and following much the same lines, but designed for use with bashful, withdrawn or disabled children. There is no need for the child to talk, his answers being limited to pointing. Obviously it is easier than the first verbal comprehension tests.

3. Expressive language, again divided into three sections depending on the child's age. At first the germs of language are explored, then the ability to name things and say what words mean, and finally the child's ability to say what he means.

The test materials are such as are likely to interest a child: toy animals, dolls, furniture and cutlery are used as the stimuli. A special section is devoted to children who are hard of hearing; scales enabling the tester to check the child's performance against the normal range are available. This test gives a good indication of a child's stage of language development in the pre-school period.

ITPA

101 The Illinois Test of Psycholinguistic Ability (ITPA) has also been revised since it was first produced, when it was intended to bridge the gap between the psychologist's and the speech therapist's areas of concern. But it is a test that is not confined to heard and spoken language. Examination of visual skills takes up half the time. An occupational therapist is fruitfully used when called in to observe this part of the lengthy test being administered.

The test sees the speech therapist as particularly interested in language development at three levels:

1. channels of communication, auditory and vocal;
2. psychological processes: the receptive, organizing and expressive processes;
3. levels of organization: automatic and representative.

There are twelve sub-tests altogether, measuring auditory and visual performance at the three levels described above. Scores for each sub-test are expressed as equivalent to a chronological age. So a graph line called a profile, linking the various sub-test scores, may show a child to be up to average for his chronological age in visual skills, but in advance or not up to his age in auditory–verbal skills – or vice versa. There may also be a wide scatter of scores which, together with findings from other tests, may suggest various causations and prognoses. The scores on the sub-tests can be consolidated into a composite psycholinguistic age, rather like the figure for a full scale IQ [67]. This is not really useful if the particular strengths and weaknesses of a child are being investigated in order to be built on or got round. The norms for the test are American, for children aged two to ten.

ITPA visual sequential memory sub-test

From the teacher's point of view the most interesting sub-test is the one for visual sequential memory. In it a child is shown a sequence of letter-like patterns and is allowed five seconds to examine them. The sequence is then withdrawn and the child has to re-create it with small tiles, each engraved with one of the letter-like patterns. Only the tiles necessary for the pattern are available. Depending on his performance with a succession of these patterns, the child is said to have a visual sequential memory – VSM for short – equivalent to a particular chronological age – from three to ten years and six months. Development of the VSM may be delayed in some cases, but often catches up at a later date, after transfer to secondary school.

This is relevant because research in the United States suggests that performance in the VSM sub-test relates closely to spelling performance. The authors' experience generally supports these findings, with these qualifications:

1. A child whose VSM development lags may be ready to learn spelling at a time when it is no longer routinely taught; more importantly, he will be at an age when much more absorbing learning experiences take up his time and attention.

2. A low VSM allied to a low average IQ will make reading progress very slow, especially at the start.

3. VSM thirty-six months below chronological age, or below 10-06 if the child is older than ten years and six months, will make good spelling impossible. Forget it, and devote the time so gained to improving spoken language, including the use of a tape recorder and telephone; woodwork; or any other skill the child enjoys. In the short term temper, and in the long term earning potential, are likely to improve.

Language tests in school

Ready-made tests for use by teachers

103 The class teacher may wonder whether a child's speech and language are such as to warrant referral to a speech therapist. Inevitably some children are borderline cases and the teacher may reasonably opt for a wait-and-see strategy, trying to rectify what she believes to be at fault and prepared to shift her ground if things do not get better.

During this period the teacher still has to identify precisely how the child is using language. She can do this in several ways: she can use ready-made tests, she can construct her own, or she can use structured observation over a period. In each case meticulous record-keeping is essential, so that the development, or lack of it, of the child's language skills over the period can be documented. If the child is eventually referred to the speech therapist, such records will provide the continuum into which the expert's view will be fitted.

The Milan Token Test checks a child's ability to understand instructions. After making sure that he is not colour blind [41] twenty coloured shapes are laid out in front of the child: five large circles, five large squares, five small circles, five small squares, each set containing one red, one blue, one white, one green and one yellow. The child is then given a series of instructions of increasing complexity: 'Show me a red one,' 'Show me the large red circle,' 'Show me the large white circle and the small green square.' At different ages the child should be able to cope with differing amounts of information requiring action. A below-average result may indicate more than just poor comprehension when other test results are taken into account.

The British Picture Vocabulary Scale (which in the United States is called the Peabody Picture Vocabulary Test – Revised) originated in America and has been adapted for use in Great Britain. It measures the heard, that is, the receptive, vocabulary of a child. The tester puts a plate with four little line drawings in front of the child and asks him to point to one in response to one stimulus word. The brevity of the stimulus limits the task to word–picture association. So this is not a test of intelligence, although it assesses one important contributor to measures of intelligence. Exposure to standard English or other cultural influences markedly affect performance. The results of this test are as useful to the teacher as to the child, for she can match her language of instruction to his level of comprehension.

The Schuell test of short-term auditory memory requires the child to repeat increasingly long series of numbers immediately after the tester has said them. Starting with two, up to seven digits are proffered. The test assesses listening skill rather than language development. Failure to complete the test satisfactorily may be associated with failure in the longer sections of the Milan Token Test, because in both the child is unable to cope with strings of words containing too much (for him) heard information.

In tests of auditory discrimination, the child has to listen to pairs of words which are either the same, 'swim – swim', or different in one particular only 'pat – bat', and the child has to say which they are. Assuming the child understands 'same' and 'different', which not all the younger ones do, his method of coping is as interesting as the score because the test is administered without the child seeing the tester's mouth. If the tester holds a card in front of her mouth, is the child trying to look round it, or asking her to repeat the pairs? Significantly, the Domain test of auditory discrimination is part of a phonic workshop, a series of worksheets teaching the early stages of reading and spelling on a direct sound–symbol association basis. There is a very good test (Bradley) which aims to find out whether a child can distinguish similarities and differences between words he hears only. Competence with this form of auditory organization is necessary for progress with both reading and spelling.

Test batteries for use by teachers

A number of publishers produce test batteries, a dozen or so tests in one package, intended to assess the skills necessary for reading. Beside auditory discrimination, auditory blending also comes up. The child hears two-, three-, four- or five-letter sounds and has to say them as a whole word, as in i-t, m-o-p, v-e-s-t, s-p-e-n-d. Again the style of response is important, but in this case the skill can be taught, and if hearing is intact, taught very successfully.

In Great Britain one of the popular test batteries is the Aston Index; this is designed to focus attention on aspects of the child's skills

104

which are important for written language. Depending on the child's age, four or five sub-tests investigate general underlying ability and attainment, and another seven or nine deal with performance. Vocabulary, auditory sequential memory, sound blending and sound discrimination are the auditory–language areas investigated for all age groups, as well as five other aspects of reading and spelling attainment. Scores on the sub-tests are plotted on to two profile sheets, the first for general underlying ability, the second for performance scores and norms. This enables the teachers to make two comparisons: (a) between the individual child's general attainments and literacy ability on the one hand and his performance on the other; and (b) between his performance (for instance on a sub-test of auditory sequential memory) and the average performance for his age group.

Structured observation

105 A teacher may, wisely, prefer to rely on observation over a period, as distinct from tests done at a particular time. Her rationale is as follows: a test of, for instance, auditory discrimination carried out in the regulated circumstances of a hospital, a health centre, or even in a quiet corner at school, will give results that scarcely show up the child's difficulty with hearing accurately in the hubbub of the classroom. And she is concerned with his performance in the classroom. In this respect London teachers have for several years been extremely well served by two systems of structured observation: Classroom Observation Procedure (COP) for children in the six plus to seven plus age range, and Development of Reading and Related Skills (DORRS) for use with children of about eleven, although literacy attainment rather than chronological age is the determinant. Both systems rely on examining what the child can do and does do from one day to the next over several weeks. Both result in detailed profiles of strengths and weaknesses seen in a context of developing literacy; both lead directly to guidance for the teacher on what and how to teach, how to organize the classroom and how to keep records of progress. The COP and DORRS checklists summarizing the teacher's knowledge of the child are the most valuable information that a teacher, worried about a pupil, can pass on to the specialist (in this case the speech therapist) called in to help.

Psychologists and speech tests

106 To some extent the clinical or educational psychologist will overlap into the speech therapist's field, certainly on the diagnostic side, though it would be a rash psychologist who embarked on giving speech therapy to a language-impaired child. Recently the British Ability Scales have been produced for use exclusively in the United Kingdom. Seven processes are tested: speed of information-processing, reasoning, spatial imagery, perceptual matching, short-term memory, retrieval and application of knowledge. The last section is directly concerned with language development. Of the six sub-tests in it, five (naming vocabulary, verbal comprehension, verbal fluency, word definitions and even word reading) are obviously an overlap into the speech therapy field. One difference lies in the fact that the scores obtained may be used to estimate an IQ rather than to identify a particular problem which needs treatment by speech therapists.

Teachers dealing with language-impaired children are well served by being given some indication of the figure for speed of information-processing.

Doctors using speech tests

As far as the medical profession is concerned, most doctors working in the field of child development in Great Britain use Mary Sheridan's Stycar kit, very fortunately often available in health clinics. It provides a rough-and-ready screen of hearing, language, vision and motor development of children. The language test is appropriate for children aged from one to seven. Common objects, miniature toys and picture books are used to find out about the child's ability to understand and express himself, using both spoken language and mime, together with symbols, such as models and pictures.

107

Summary (98–103)

The speech therapist deals with development of language. This has become far more important than her old role of curing stammers and stutters.

She can tell you if your child's language has not developed properly. She can also tell you if he is not good at listening.

She may give him speech therapy. She may tell you and his teacher how to improve his language and listening skills.

Quite often she needs to go into the classroom to listen to your child in an everyday setting.

Some of her tests are the same as those used by the psychologists, but the two test different aspects of language.

Chapter Ten
Threats to Brain Function

Introduction

The neurons [52], the brain's main cells, are very vulnerable to lack of oxygen, physical damage, biochemical disturbances and a variety of poisons. They are most susceptible when in a growing phase. Once dead they cannot be replaced, though early on in life their functions may be taken over by other brain cells. Fortunately there are thousands of them, so we can afford to lose a lot and hardly notice anything amiss.

A number of substances and types of injury are known to cause damage to the brain cells. The extent and the effects depend not only on the intensity of the insult but also on the stage of development of the brain at the time the incident occurs and on the individuality of the child.

Some of the more frequently discussed conditions have been arranged chronologically, that is, in an order relating to the stages of development of the child.

Genetic possibilities

108 Boys have a higher incidence of learning disabilities than girls, so sex may play a part. Learning disabilities run in families, so perhaps they are inherited. Is dyslexia of genetic origin?

Our inherited characteristics are carried by genes lying on twenty-three pairs of chromosomes, rod-like structures found in the nuclei of our cells. The ovum and the sperm each contribute only one chromosome to each pair, so the baby gets characteristics from both parents, at least as far as twenty-two out of the twenty-three pairs are concerned. In the male, one pair is made up of the X and the Y chromosomes, the former being larger than the latter. In women, the pair is made of two X chromosomes. Each chromosome coming from a different parent, this X and Y system is responsible for the sex of the baby. But from the time the midwife says, 'It's a boy', knitting needles are shrouded in blue wool and social factors also play a part in determining masculinity. By the time he or she is eighteen months old, the toddler has a pretty good idea whether he or she is meant to be a boy or a girl. The full chain develops: chromosomes – anatomy – social mores – puberty – reproductive capability.

It is tempting to think that somewhere in the X and Y system there are genes which determine reading ability, or a lack of it. As yet there is no positive proof of the existence of such a gene. What is known is that the small male Y chromosome seems to carry little except genes which determinine masculinity. The large female X chromosome does have other attributes not directly related to femininity. On the surface, these do not seem to be directly related to learning disabilities. Sensitivity to Vitamin D, the volume of urine passed, susceptibility to some drug-induced anaemias, upsets in clotting, colour vision, calcium metabolism attributes, and some of the defences against bacteriological infections are carried by genes lying on the X chromosome, of which the woman has two and the man only one. What the relationship, if any, is between the genes determining sex and dyslexia is not known. The only well-established fact is that there are more boys with learning disabilities than girls with those problems.

Some of us are unfortunate enough to be born with the wrong ration of X or Y chromosomes. This is a very rare occurrence. There are two patterns which are sometimes not recognized early and are mistaken for cases of specific developmental dyslexia.

Boys may have an extra chromosome, so that the pattern is X X Y, instead of the normal X Y. Such children have abnormalities of hormone production, may be mentally retarded but are not necessarily so, and cannot have children when they grow up. Though some are anti-social, others are placid and biddable, easy to have at home. They do not do well at school and may have difficulty in learning to read. Some respond symptomatically to hormone treatment and become rough, tough, active boys with concomitant improvement in their reading. Not all mothers welcome the change and in some instances have been known to reject therapy, letting their child revert to the happy, placid state.

On the distaff side, similar disturbances in genetic make-up may occur. A girl with only one X chromosome will be small, with a thick-set neck. She will not be able to have babies when she grows up. This condition is called Turner's syndrome after the doctor who first described it in 1938. Most children with this condition do badly in the performance part of the W I S C-R I Q test [69], may not be much good at maths and have difficulty with right/left discrimination [79]. Perhaps the right half of the brain is not functioning as well as it should [56]. The child health clinic should spot these cases and most are identified early. There is no cure and no known way of preventing these sad cases.

Robin's family had come from another English-speaking country, where she had been to school in a remote area with few medical facilities. She entered the English school system when she was almost ten. After a couple of terms, she was referred to the educational psychologist because she presented what her form teacher called an unusual picture. Apparently she talked rapidly and indistinctly, frequently stopping a sentence in mid-flow and re-starting in an effort to get her message across.

The educational psychologist found that she was generally bright, but thought that there might be some underlying physical disorder and had her referred to the hospital because she was so small. She came to the clinic via the paediatrician who had made a tentative diagnosis of Turner's syndrome, which was later confirmed.

When first seen, her handwriting was legible but she found it difficult to do. She had very great difficulty in recalling sequences of digits [102] and it certainly was difficult to understand her when she spoke. The speech therapist established that her expressive language was rapid with frequent telescoping of multisyllabic words and that she left out the small parts of speech, like 'a', 'the', 'it', 'so' and 'up'. Frequently she only achieved an approximation of the sound at which she was aiming. The speech therapist felt that there was a problem [98] which could be helped by her therapy. The occupational therapist identified a similar problem, for which she too could offer therapy.

Turner's syndrome is a rarity – a lot of doctors will go through their professional lives without ever seeing one case. Robin's case does show the need for a child to be seen by a paediatrician early on, if things are not going well. Geography and circumstances do not always allow of such luxury.

Summary (108)

Learning disabilities are commoner in some families than in others.

More boys have learning disabilities than girls.

There is a strong suspicion that a genetic element causes learning disabilities.

No positive proof has been found that learning disabilities are inherited.

No reason for the high incidence of boys with learning disabilities is known.

Alcohol taken in pregnancy

109

If a mother drinks a great deal of alcohol during the course of her pregnancy, the risk of damage to the baby is high. If she has only an occasional drink during the week, no need to worry. Fortunately, most women go off drink when pregnant, so nature is its own watchdog. If you like a lot to drink and intend to become or suddenly find yourself pregnant, do consult your family doctor. Do not panic or feel conscience-stricken if you went to a good party and then found yourself pregnant. The danger is the regular intake of alcohol.

High alcohol intake can result in the baby being born with the 'foetal alcohol syndrome'. The child has a hairy face, a poorly formed upper jaw, sometimes a cleft palate or heart trouble, and often some degree of mental retardation. The clinical picture is very obvious. The mental retardation is usually only slight and most children can cope with ordinary school. There may be some lack of coordination which interferes with fine hand-skills.

This danger is easy to avoid by considerably reducing a high alcohol intake. In simple language, do not drink a lot when pregnant.

Rubella and the pregnant mother

110

Rubella (German measles) contracted by a pregnant woman may cause blindness, deafness and congenital heart disease in the baby she is carrying. It may also result in mild brain damage and learning disabilities when the child reaches school age.

Nowadays it is quite unnecessary to get rubella when pregnant. Those of us who develop German measles in childhood have a natural immunity against further attacks. However, there are other virus diseases which produce a very similar picture in the sufferer and it may be difficult to know whether the rash is or is not due to rubella. You will meet people who are convinced that they have had two attacks of

German measles. They haven't; they have had two different diseases. All schoolgirls are, or should be, checked to make sure that they have adequate natural immunity against the disease. If they are found to be susceptible, then they should be immunized. Even when this has been done, it is still important to get your rubella status checked if you are thinking about having a baby. If you have not enough protection then you can be immunized, but not after you have started the baby. Prevention is simple. Make sure you are protected and your baby will be safe.

Although the ill-effects of rubella are well known, precise information about the results of other virus infections affecting the mother during pregnancy is lacking. There are times when doctors are reasonably sure that such an infection has affected the baby, but have no positive proof. Take the case of Arthur, for instance.

During her pregnancy, Arthur's mother had a severe virus infection affecting the lining of her brain. She was very ill during the whole of the sixth month.

The delivery was about three weeks late and the baby weighed 8 lbs 9 oz. He was difficult to feed and was a restless, unsatisfied baby. He was very floppy, late in learning to sit up and did not walk until he was twenty months. He had also a wry neck and his testes did not come down unaided but had to be put in the scrotum surgically.

At school he was slow to learn, and his appalling handwriting was a constant source of friction between him and his teacher. He was quite good at reading.

When he came to the clinic at the age of eleven he was a bit of a loner and was always in trouble at school, where he was teased a lot. He was no good at outdoor games, but enjoyed chess. He was well aware of his problems.

His coordination was very poor and he showed a lot of excessive movements, so much so that, when testing his language development, the speech therapist had to ask him to sit on his hands as they distracted both him and her. His tongue movements were what she termed 'dyspraxic': there was no paralysis but he could not make his tongue do what he wanted it to.

His IQ was average, but this disguised the fact that his verbal IQ was 120 (superior) and his performance IQ 96 [68, 69].

He was taught to write using only his hand and wrist; before, his elbow had joined in the process. The occupational therapist saw him regularly and improved his coordination.

The last we heard from him was that he was taking O-levels, but we never learnt the results. We hope that this means he got the exam results he wanted. He had been told that, if all did not go well, he could receive a recommendation from the clinic to the Examining Board for special consideration in view of the medical nature of his condition. That he did not ask for this was, we felt, a good sign.

Lead and the pregnant mother

Lead has been recognized as a poison for years: at one time it was used to produce abortions. It can get into the body in different ways. If heated to over 500°C – hotter than melted solder – it gives off fumes which may be breathed in. If ground up finely, it can be inhaled as dust or can contaminate food and cigarettes from the fingers. The lead in petrol can be absorbed directly through the skin, and, when the petrol is burnt, the lead can get into the atmosphere. It can find its way into drinking water from old-fashioned lead pipes if the local water is 'soft' – that is, on the acid side.

The principal risks of exposure for adults occur at work, so there are stringent regulations to minimize the chances of lead being absorbed. In the United Kingdom, a Code of Practice for the Control of Lead at Work has been drawn up by the Health and Safety Executive and is obtainable from H.M. Stationery Office. All types of hazardous work-processes are listed, and there are details of control measures and of the medical monitoring necessary to ensure the safety of the worker. There is a special section about women exposed to lead at work; it is necessary that women should be exposed to lower levels of lead than men.

Extra care is needed to ensure that an unborn child is not put at risk. Lead crosses the placental barrier and passes from the mother's blood to the baby; this must not be allowed to happen. If the foetus is exposed to lead, the effects may be either immediate or delayed. It is thought that small quantities have a damaging effect on developing nerve cells and that learning disabilities may result in later life. However, the direct connection between lead absorbed across the placenta and poor reading or spelling six or more years later has not been firmly established. The difficulty in reaching a firm conclusion lies in the speed with which lead may leave the body or be deposited in the bones. All of us carry a small amount, whether we are lead workers, live near a lead smelter, work in a pay-booth in an indoor car park, or just live in an urban or near-urban environment. Exposure to lead at work will push up our blood lead levels, but so may some do-it-yourself activities.

A pregnant woman busy nesting may unwittingly put herself and her baby at risk. The Victorians in the last century used lead in paint to give it a longer life and lead may be found all over an old house: in some wallpapering, as a filler in wood where a chisel may have slipped, anywhere where there is paint. Old cots and banisters may be sanded down to show the natural wood, and you, a mother-to-be, may be raising a cloud of lead dust with your electrical machine. You can breathe this dust in, or get it on your food, your teacup or your cigarette. Before you start work with the sander on an old painted surface, ask the local Environmental Health Officer if he thinks there could be anything to worry about. He will be able to advise you.

How much lead can be tolerated without damage to the baby? The answer is not clearly known. The direct correlation between lead in the air and blood lead levels is recognized when it comes to the upper safety limits and you will find these in the Code of Practice. What is not certain is how much lead is safe, from a baby's point of view. So to be on the safe side, if you work with lead, ask your family doctor – or perhaps the firm's doctor – if you should have a check of your blood lead levels early on in pregnancy.

But frankly, the chances of you or your baby being poisoned by lead are small.

Summary (111)
Too much lead is bad for you and your unborn baby.
You can be at risk if you work with lead.
If your job exposes you to a significant amount of lead, you should be monitored by your firm's doctor.
If you burn or scrape off old lead paint when redecorating your home, you could be exposed to lead fumes or dust.
Ask the local Environmental Health Officer if you are worried about this.
Lead poisoning is a very rare disease.

The hazards of being born

112 It used to be said that the most dangerous thing a man ever did was to be born. Nowadays the risks of being damaged during birth have been reduced to a minimum. The activities of the doctors, midwives and anaesthetists around the time of the happy event are directed towards ensuring a safe delivery. Even so, on rare occasions things may not go according to plan.

Obvious neurological conditions, such as cerebral palsy, may result from a reduction of blood supply to the brain; trauma may cause what is in effect a stroke; too much bile pigment, making the baby very jaundiced, may do harm. A lot of babies are a bit yellow on arrival, but this passes off quickly and is of no consequence. Too little sugar in the blood or an inbalance of various salts may be harmful.

All these possibilities are recognized by doctors and the baby is watched so that, if anything untoward happens, steps can be taken to avoid trouble. In general, it is agreed that severe damage with obvious neurological change will result in learning disabilities later. What is not so certain is the connection between minimal brain damage and learning disabilities [136]. The sort of evidence which supports that possibility is statistical. A few years ago, babies of low birth weight stood a good chance of developing learning disabilities later, if they survived the initial few weeks of life. Now improved methods of premature-baby care have reduced the damaging effects of nutritional and biochemical hazards and there has been a marked improvement in their long-term outlook, with much less chance of learning disabilities.

A baby who has suffered some untoward event around the time of his birth should be regarded as being at greater risk of having a learning disability, but not as an inevitable candidate for the remedial class. There is an increased chance, but certainly no certainty of problems in school. A poor language environment [86], family stress [127], glue ears [32] or head injuries [119] may supervene. For the neurologically intact baby who has had an uneventful birth, the chances of his overcoming handicaps of childhood are greater than they are for his less fortunate cousin who was blue from lack of oxygen or white from shock on arrival in this world.

Parents should be aware that different sorts of specialists emphasize different sorts of 'at risk' factors. Sociologists see family economics and social opportunity as vital, the psychologists stress family dynamics, doctors regard physical factors as important. We are all hucksters of our own wares. The child can be viewed from one angle only, but the risks which may threaten a child are many and all types must be considered when trying to find out why a child is failing to learn to read or spell.

It is cheering that the number of children at risk through medical factors is falling dramatically and that modern medical care is so effective in curtailing the chances of learning disabilities developing later. It is important to attend the antenatal clinic and the child development clinic so that your baby can have the best possible start in life.

Angus was tiny when born – he weighed 2 lbs – and he stayed in hospital, receiving the very best of care, until he was three months old. Then the paediatrician kept a close eye on him until he was four.

As a baby he had been a bit uncoordinated; when a little older he had difficulty in putting food into his mouth, and much later on he could not use a knife. He was six before he managed to put his shoes on by himself. Drawing skills took a long time to come and at nursery school he was the only child who never managed to do a 'painting'. Though very courageous, he never really learnt to swim because his arms and legs would not work in unison. Ball games were a disaster, but he always went on trying.

His reading and spelling were excellent and he was distinctly bright. His only real problem was his handwriting, which was slow, laborious and not joined up. When seen in the clinic at the age of ten and a half, he was well adjusted, cheerful, chatty and fully aware of his difficulties. His Neale test [165] scores were: reading comprehension age level, twelve years and four months; reading accuracy, eleven years and eleven months; speed, adult. His silent reading comprehension in the Gapadol test [166] was above the adult level and his spelling was a year in advance of his age. To help his handwriting, the occupational therapist gave him a special programme [186, 187, 189, 190, 191] in the holidays, he was encouraged to use a Pentel pen or a well-sharpened pencil and he was shown how to put letters with descenders (f, g, j, p, q, y) correctly on the line. He was told not to hold the pen so tightly and to try not to rest his head on his left hand while writing.

At the end of the summer holidays, he was producing a non-cursive, difficult-to-read scrawl. The ascenders and descenders were not long enough and he had a purely individualistic way of forming lots of letters, for instance 𝒶 for 'a', the pen going clockwise.

So he attended the Occupational Therapy Department

twice a week for a month, worked his way through pre-writing exercises [189] and progressed to proper cursive writing.

By the end of the term, his pencil grip was still too tight and his writing slow. But he knew what he had to do to improve, and he had got the ascenders and descenders more in proportion.

Five months later, the occupational therapist got an ecstatic telephone call to say that he had been accepted by an academic school of his and his parents' choice. There was joy all round and the new school never made a murmur about his handwriting.

Minor brain damage

Major brain damage, from whatever causes, produces easily recognizable after-effects. Educational problems can be anticipated and help organized at an early stage. Between such important disasters and that shadowy entity 'minimal brain dysfunction' [136] lies a wide variety of conditions in which the damage is minor but definite. The affected child may progress through early life supported and encouraged by his family, who are not aware that anything is seriously amiss – 'Johnny has always had a lopsided smile', 'I have always thought that Sharon's left leg was a bit shorter than her right', 'Harry was late to talk, but then his sisters always answered for him.'

When the demands of school have to be met, the perceptual or language problems secondary to the underlying minor brain damage become apparent. Clinical examination of these children reveals definite physical signs to the doctor (not 'soft' ones [136]). Special investigations confirm that there is something wrong. One cerebral hemisphere (often the right one) may be smaller than the other. The brain tissue may have shrunk a little, or perhaps the ventricle, the fluid-filled space inside [50] may be larger on one side than the other.

Brain scans, electroencephalograms [121] or other painless investigations are used to reach a diagnosis. The psychologist's tests [67] may identify the perceptual mechanism at fault. The doctor may be able to give a prognosis, so that the future limitations of the child can be determined. Teachers can be told of the child's inevitable weaknesses and of his strengths so that appropriate classroom techniques can be used. The parents can understand the child's problems and recognize both his limitations and his potential. It helps to know what is hap-

113

pening, and why. But remember, the diagnosis can be made only by a doctor.

Jimmy had had a stormy birth: his mother's labour was long, he was a big baby, weighing over 9 lbs, and forceps had to be used. He had to be cot-nursed for a few days. He was difficult to feed at first and did not suck well. Later he was slow to walk, getting going on his own at about eighteen months. He had no difficulty with talking and was always chatty. Photographs of him as a toddler showed that he had a slightly lopsided smile.

He was not particularly clumsy, just not very handy. He used his right hand in preference to his left. His mother remarked spontaneously that he almost needed a larger size of shoe on his right foot than on his left. He is, she said, very right-sided. She was correct. No, he never enjoyed jig-saw puzzles. By the time he got to school, he was a cheerful, outgoing boy. But he was very slow to learn to read. He could not master the letters and never recognized word shapes. His cheerfulness began to wear thin.

The psychologist found that he had a normal IQ (WISC-R full scale 109 [67]) but this hid a significant discrepancy between the verbal IQ score of 113 and the performance IQ score of 89 [70]. His block design score was particularly low [69].

The speech therapist found nothing wrong with his language except that he was a little 'dyspraxic', by which she meant that he had difficulty in getting his tongue round words.

He could barely read and his spelling was completely disorganized. The doctor found that he was certainly lopsided. His skull was larger on the left than the right, his smile was crooked and his tongue protruded slightly to the right. There were other signs that suggested a very minor form of stroke affecting the left side of his body.

Brain scanning and an electroencephalogram confirmed that he had a large ventricle [50] on the right side of his cerebrum, with consequent reduction in the amount of brain tissue in the right cerebral hemisphere. This was not enough damage to make him disfigured or disabled, but enough to reduce the normal functioning of that half of the brain. He had difficulty in coping with shapes and with look-and-say reading techniques [57]. There was an imbalance between the left and right cerebral hemispheres and nothing anybody could do would alter that. However, he had great strengths on the verbal side.

Recognition of his problem eased expectation from adults so that his tension lessened. Special teaching programmes using his verbal strengths were recommended, but there was no disguising the fact that it was going to be an uphill battle for everyone.

To sum up, he had minor brain damage which handicapped but did not disable him, in a physical sense anyway.

John was a big baby – 10 lb 2 oz at birth. For the first few months he was so drowsy that his mother used to wake him up to see if he was alive. She did this in spite of having had three children before him.

When he was three he had a febrile convulsion. An electroencephalogram at the time suggested that the attack was epileptic and might therefore recur, so he was put on phenobarbitone for two years. His left foot was turned in and this was thought to be due to a mild cerebral palsy – a corrective operation set it right. He never got on well at school, but initially the parents were told to wait. By the time he was seven the school was anxious too and he was given remedial help twice a week to improve his reading.

He came to the clinic when he was eleven. His parents said he was a loner, but happy. He was no good at games, but enjoyed swimming. His mother had noticed that he sometimes lost himself while watching T V. To meet, he was chatty and informative. He had great difficulty in recalling specific names – he could not say where his older married brother lived, he did not know the name of the book he was reading and he did not know the months of the year. His Neale test scores [165] were all at the seven years and six months level and his Schonell spelling test scores [173] at the five years and eight months level. When reading the Neale text, he would read each passage carefully to himself before he read it aloud and he would often substitute wrong words. When it came to the comprehension questions he answered them correctly, using the written word in his reply and not his substituted one.

An electroencephalogram showed a generalized abnormality compatible with minimal brain damage at birth. There was no sign of epilepsy. The clinical psychologist found his verbal IQ to be 92, his performance IQ to be 111 and the full scale WISC-RIQ to be 101. She remarked that he was inattentive, needed instructions to be repeated and chattered away incessantly. His lowest score was in the general information sub-test [68], which was understandable since he had never read for fun. Interestingly enough, he was unable to name the shop in which sugar is bought, and then added that he called those shops 'ardens'. When asked about the meaning of this, he shrugged and said it wasn't a proper word but that it was *his* word for that kind of shop. In contrast, his verbal reasoning was well above average.

Clinically, he had slight but positive signs of a weakness and he was left-handed.

The somewhat diffuse picture which he presented, with enough physical signs to make the doctors sure that he had neurological abnormalities, is typical of minor as opposed to minimal [136] brain damage. The long-term educational prospects were not good.

114 Too much calcium

There is a very rare condition which occurs during the late months of pregnancy or in early infancy. The child has too much calcium, the main constituent of chalk and bones, in his body. A neurological disturbance results, with a reduction in the number of neurons (nerve cells). Between the third and seventh months after birth the infant suddenly fails to thrive. At this stage the condition is usually reversible. If severe and unchecked, the child may develop a smaller-than-usual head, an 'elfin' face, a heart murmur and some degree of mental retardation. If the condition is mild, the diagnosis may not be considered until the child reaches school. Modern methods of infant supervision usually ensure that the condition is identified early, so go to the child development clinic when given an appointment. If your three-month-old baby is not doing well, do not rely on the neighbours for advice; tell the doctor.

Annette was referred to the hospital by her family doctor because she was doing badly at school. She was said to have

poor concentration, temper tantrums, and to be always running
to the lavatory. At home her behaviour was better, provided
that she had the undivided attention of an adult. This was the
usual picture of a dyslexic child. Her story was that in early
childhood she had slept very badly and did not do well in the
first six months, otherwise she had an uneventful medical
history, or so it seemed.

She did not resemble either her father or her mother, who
both came to the clinic with her. On direct questioning, it
seemed that she did not look like anyone else in the family
either.

She had a very small head for her age (seven years
exactly), her bite was not very good – her teeth did not meet
effectively – and she was certainly very active, distractable and
difficult to pin down to any task. Her IQ was low average
(WISC-R verbal IQ, 83; performance IQ, 95) and her sub-test
scores were patchy. The psychologist thought the uneven
scores were most likely due to her fluctuating concentration,
but she did seem to have some problem with visual perception.
In fact her reading was within normal limits for her age, though
she had great difficulty in spelling even her own name. During
all the tests she kept up a flood of conversation and was very
fidgety.

She was referred to the child psychiatrist and the
consultant paediatrician who had a clinic together, and the latter
considered her to be a case of ideopathic (i.e. of unknown
origin) hypercalcaemia, that is, too much chalk in infancy.

The clinic has only seen two cases of this rare condition.
The lesson for parents lies in her odd appearance. There are
many medical reasons why children should not look like anyone
else in a family, so this clue should always be followed up.

Allergies

We are allergic if the body's normal protective systems go wrong so
that what should be a defensive reaction to something turns out to be
harmful. Asthma, eczema and hay fever are the three principal allergic
reactions, but there can be less obvious or dramatic symptoms. Food
additives have long been suspected of causing hyperactivity in some
children, with inattentiveness and poor school performance as a result.

115

THREATS TO BRAIN FUNCTION

It is not easy to pinpoint the actual substance with accuracy. The paediatrician must exclude the commoner causes for hyperkinesis [134] first. If the doctor feels that there are grounds for incriminating food additives, then he will probably recommend a trial period during which many foods containing colouring matter or artificial flavourings are avoided.

Parents should not attempt such dietary restrictions on their own and should always seek professional advice. To limit your child's diet on vague suspicion is to run the risk of producing a dietary deficiency of some sort. You may starve him accidentally. Never be too much of a disciplinarian about food restrictions; any normal child strays from the narrow path of dietary righteousness from time to time. Imposition of strict food laws may result in anorexia nervosa, a self-imposed starvation of much greater importance than being a poor speller.

Brain infections

116 Surprisingly enough, generalized brain infections or brain fevers such as meningitis or encephalitis do not usually produce learning disabilities. There was an epidemic years ago which did receive some publicity because attacks of encephalitis were followed by classroom problems, but it is rarely seen these days. If Granny tells you about children she went to school with who had problems after brain fevers, agree with her, but do not worry on your child's account. However, some common or garden virus infections such as measles may very occasionally lead to later learning disabilities. Part of the controversy surrounding immunization against whooping cough has centred round the relative risks of getting brain damage from the disease or from the protective injection. The general rule is to get your child immunized against as many diseases as are common to the country in which you live. Always consult your doctor just before this is done; there are some children who should not receive immunization.

In summary, avoidance of disease is part of the prevention of dyslexia.

Poisoning and children

117 All sorts of substances are beneficial in small doses and harmful if taken in excess.

Poisoning may occur for a number of reasons. Something may be swallowed when its correct use does not include absorption into the human body. An overdose of medicine may turn a useful drug into a dangerous one. Some poisons may be taken for their stimulating effects.

On the whole, it is the toddler or the child who has just gone to school who is most likely to swallow something he shouldn't, mistaking it for something else. Children manage to take a wide range of things, from paraffin (kerosene) to their mother's contraceptives. The rescue operation always involves consideration of the long-term outlook and if there is a possibility of learning disability later on, as the result of the toxic effects, the doctor should let you know. Doctor-induced effects – called iatrogenic disease – can result from poor communication between parents and doctors or from the overall ignorance of the potency of some substance. An overdose resulting from parents doubling the pre-scribed amount of anti-epileptic drugs is an example of the first. Un-derstandably, parents are fearful of epileptic fits occurring to their child once they have seen him have one. When they think that a convulsion might be coming on, perhaps because of a fever, they double the usual dose of the drug and continue this increased dose for some time. Pheny-toin is associated with learning disabilities [122] and needs careful medical control. The thalidomide disaster is the outstanding example of the result of general ignorance of the potency of some chemicals. Knowledge came too late for some. Always ask your doctor about the possible side-effects of medicines.

In the United Kingdom, the Poisons Bureau will respond rapidly to requests for information from your doctor or the casualty officer should there be doubt about what your child has taken, what the effects are and what antidote applies. If the poisoning is by some industrial chemical, the Employment Medical Advisory Service of the Health and Safety Executive can also give information about the effects. What is much more difficult to identify are the drugs children take for fun. In London, alcohol still rates high among favourite forms of self-poisoning. It is easy for a gang of youngsters to raid a supermarket and come away with flat bottles of booze.

Glue and other solvents, cannabis, heroin, amphetamines, and combinations of these, may be used. So what are the indications that your son is exploring illicit possibilities? A falling-off of performance and of behaviour in a child who has hitherto kept a steady profile is often the first clue. The learning-disabled, with all the misery and frustrations that go with poor school performance, are particularly vulnerable to drug abuse. There is nothing like a quick sniff to make your troubles vanish. The educational psychologist may find a much lower IQ than previous testings recorded. This should always be a reason for further investigation. Never reject an IQ because it does not tally with one done some years back. It is disheartening to be suddenly told that your child is not as bright as you thought he was, but the change may be due to an underlying medical condition. It does not have to be drugs; it could even be something simple, like glandular fever. Get him checked.

It is sometimes difficult to know whether the learning disability is the reason why a child resorts to drugs or whether his addiction runs in parallel with his school failure.

Tim's parents were both self-employed. He was born normally and was a cuddly, easy baby. He suffered a lot of middle-ear disease between the ages of three months and four years [31].

It was not until his second year at school that things began to go wrong. Boisterous, tough, athletic, with lots of friends, by the age of nine he could only read at the six years and eight months level. His spelling was at the six-year mark. His IQ was in the low average range (WISC-R verbal IQ, 92; performance IQ, 82; full scale IQ, 86). His auditory and visual sequential memories [73, 102] were at the six-year level. His understanding and expression of language were limited. So far, par for the course for a child with low average intelligence and early ear trouble. He got lots of extra help, with benefit. Then, three years after first being seen, his behaviour began to deteriorate. He stopped attending clubs, he opted out of the football team, he exposed himself in the street and he began to sleep very badly. Because it was an 'in' craze for his age group, he was suspected of glue-sniffing; extensive investigations did not confirm this suspicion. He was discovered to be drinking at least four pints of strong black coffee a day – not, of course, the single reason for his changed behaviour, but a contributory factor.

Toby was born happily into his middle-class family. His parents were to divorce when he was six. At the age of three he started to have fits in association with fevers. These were controlled by phenobarbitone, which he took for about eighteen months. He did, however, have some more fits when he had chickenpox at the age of six. Investigations at the time, including an electroencephalogram, showed that he did not have epilepsy and he received no medication. He always slept badly and wet his bed until he was twelve. He had the greatest difficulty in learning to read, but was athletic, musical and good at painting and pottery. He was seen as a nice, creative boy. When his I Q was found to be in the superior range (WISC-R verbal I Q, 120; performance I Q, 135; full scale I Q, 130) he was thought to have a specific learning difficulty. He received a great deal of remedial help. By the time he was fourteen he began to truant and got into trouble for using cannabis, amphetamines and cocaine. A year later his verbal I Q was 94, his performance I Q was 107, and his full scale I Q was 100. His reading age was that of a six-year-old. He was depressed, deluded and suicidal. The learning disability was of secondary importance for this poor boy. The falling-off in his I Q scores was directly related to his drug-taking.

Lead again

Lead can be inhaled as dust or fumes, eaten if it gets on to food or our fingers, or absorbed through the skin if it is in petrol. Once in, it may affect the red pigment in blood and hence the transport of oxygen to the cells. Harmful effects of lead vary from a barely detectable drop in the amount of red-cell pigment (haemoglobin) to frank anaemia with obvious pallor and tiredness. Loss of appetite, constipation and bad stomach cramps may follow. Nerves supplying muscles may be temporarily put out of action with consequent paralysis, the kidneys may be damaged and, in extreme cases, there may be fits and loss of consciousness. The dose of lead has to be large if it is to produce these extreme effects. A rise in blood lead levels matches the increasing severity of the symptoms.

Lead intoxication of a severe sort is very rarely found in children. Minor forms may arise if the child chews something old which has been coated with lead paint – the bars of an old cot or wallpaper in an old room. Children playing illicitly on an industrial site or in a junkyard may pick up dust. Perhaps used car batteries have been broken up with axes to get at the valuable lead plates in them. Living near a polluting industrial source used to be a hazard. New legislation is directed at ensuring that the local atmosphere is not contaminated; as a consequence the risk has been reduced. Lead from the exhausts of cars using leaded petrol had been under suspicion as a source of trouble for some time.

There have been reports that children with high body burdens of lead, but without signs of lead poisoning, have lowered I Qs, are

118

hyperactive and have more learning disabilities than children with low lead levels. Urban children are known to have higher blood lead levels than country children. The fear is that the lead in the air may be causing minimal brain dysfunction and that lead-laden petrol fumes are the cause. Careful studies have had difficulty in substantiating these fears. Genetic, perinatal, nutritional, socio-economic and family factors must all be taken into account, and when they are the situation becomes less clear.

It is only too easy to assume that because a child is doing badly at school and because he is one of a group with higher-than-average levels of lead, then it is the lead which makes him overactive, badly behaved and a poor scholar. High blood lead levels may be associated with a low family income, poor surroundings and dirt. So are learning difficulties. It may be that the social conditions are the real cause, and that the lead is only a parallel symptom alongside the learning difficulties and does not cause them.

The present state of knowledge is far from satisfactory. It would be rash to assume that, if all our children's blood lead levels were very low, they would read and spell beautifully.

Nine-year-old Mary came to the clinic because her school performance had suddenly dropped off and she had begun to complain of stomach-aches every morning. To begin with these were bad enough for her to see the doctor, but he found nothing wrong. Now, it is always important to ask what a child's dad does for a living. The same goes for the mother, though it is best to find out if her job before marriage was different from that after marriage. The parents' employment can have a bearing on a case. So the mother was asked: 'What did her man do?' 'He worked for a demolition firm.' 'Yes, but doing what?' 'He cut up the steel girders when they were taking a building down.' 'Do you mean he was a burner – he used a gas cutting torch?' 'Yes, that's right.' Hot on the scent, the doctor got quite excited. 'Is it a big firm?' 'Oh no, quite a small one.' 'Who washes his overalls?' 'I do. He always brings them home and I put them in the washing machine with the other jeans and things.' A possible clue. Old steel girders are often covered in lead paint. Cutting them with a hot torch produces lead fumes and dust, which gets on the overalls and perhaps, in this case, came home with dad.

THREATS TO BRAIN FUNCTION

Could the child have a mild dose of lead poisoning? Blood tests showed that she hadn't. In fact she needed glasses, as she was short-sighted and could not see the blackboard from the back of the class. Still, it's a point to remember.

Head injuries in childhood

119

All children bang their heads hard at some time – 'Mummy, I hurted myself.' Those in their first years of school are especially prone to accidental head injuries. There are three types of damage: closed, open and minor.

A *closed head injury* is one where the skull bones are not broken. It is usually caused by a blow from a blunt object. The seriousness of the injury determines the length of time before full recovery. The longer the child is unconscious and the longer it takes for his memory for recent events to return to normal, the longer it will be before he is fully recovered. The long-term effects of a severe closed head injury include a falling-off of intellectual functioning, and bad behaviour. The child may become overactive, restless and excessively chatty. He may be aggressive, depressed and anti-social. There may be outbursts of inappropriate behaviour – undressing at the wrong time and in the wrong place, for example. Visuo-motor or visuo-spatial functions [64, 65] are usually more affected than verbal ones. If the WISC-R IQ [67] is done, there may be changes compared with a test done before the injury. Coupled with the behaviour problems, this cognitive impairment will have an adverse effect on school performance.

Recovery may be slow, depending on the severity of the injury. There is usually a steady improvement during the first year, but it may take as long as four years before everything gets back to normal. There will also be a lot of catching up. 'Getting back to normal' means back to normal functioning and not normal achievement.

An *open head injury* is one where the skull bones are broken: there is a fracture. There may be no loss of consciousness, but the injury is serious none the less. Local damage to brain tissue may occur. The after-effects differ from those of closed head injuries. The functions or sensations of a limb or part of the body may be lost. Epilepsy [120] is commoner as a late complication of open rather than closed head injuries. Doctors in charge of the child at the time of the injury should be able to give an indication not only of the immediate prospects but also of the long-term outlook.

In all cases of serious head injury, the level of the child's intelligence together with his achievements prior to the accident determine the baseline to which he can be expected to return on recovery.

Minor head injuries are those where there is no loss of consciousness, no loss of memory and no fracture of the skull. No long-lasting effects result from minor head injuries. Do not feel guilty if your baby once slipped off the bed when you were changing his nappy, hit his head and was rushed to hospital in your panic. Even if they kept him in overnight, 'just to make sure', and let him out next day, no long-lasting damage will have been done. If, six years later on, he is behind with his reading, you will have to look elsewhere for the cause.

Summary (119)

Head injuries causing loss of consciousness, loss of immediate memory for the day's events or a fractured skull may be important.

Long-term effects may be cognitive and behavioural problems.

Occasionally, epilepsy follows severe head injury.

Minor bangs on the head are of no importance.

Epilepsy

120 Epilepsy signifies spasmodic losses of consciousness due to abnormal brain activity – 'fits'. It can occur either in association with brain disease such as cerebral palsy or without any evidence of physical abnormality. Birth injuries, congenital defects, head injuries, some familial diseases causing brain degeneration, lead poisoning and tumours may all be associated with epilepsy. However, it usually happens spontaneously, with no changes in brain structure. Four main types of seizure occur in children: grand mal, petit mal, psycho-motor and focal. More than one type may occur in the same patient.

Grand mal

This is the classic form of epilepsy. Hours before the attack occurs, the child may get some warning. He may be irritable or behave in a peculiar fashion; he may complain of giddiness or of an uncomfortable stomach. These sensations are followed by the rolling upwards of the eyes, loss of consciousness and the fit itself, when the whole body is convulsed by alternate spasms and relaxation. The child may stop breathing and go blue. A seizure may vary in length from a few seconds to half an hour. Very rarely, one attack is followed by another without the child regaining consciousness in between. This rare state is an emergency and medical help should be sought immediately.

After the seizure, the child is semi-conscious and confused. If he responds to questions he will not know what he is saying. This is a general description and each child may exhibit his own variations on the main theme. Fits of any sort may be encouraged by the onset of fever, by infections, tiredness, emotional upset, flickering lights or even by the sudden withdrawal of anti-epileptic drugs. Little children may have a fever fit at the onset of an illness and this may have nothing to do with epilepsy. The general course is variable, but some children who suffer from grand mal in early childhood apparently get better and then start fits again after puberty.

Petit mal

Petit mal implies very brief losses of consciousness without convulsions. If no other types of seizure occur, it is thought that the attacks are due to overactivity in the deeper parts of the brain. Petit mal first appears in childhood, usually between five and nine years old, and is commoner among girls than boys. The onset is quick, the child suddenly developing twenty or more attacks a day. Each is a short loss of consciousness lasting up to ten seconds and coming without warning. There may be some slight twitching of the face or sucking with the lips. Recovery is quick and most patients do not realize that anything has happened. Nor may the teacher, if the condition has not been diagnosed before. Who can spot a momentary lapse of attention of one child out of a class of thirty? The results can lead anyone to think that he has just been idling.

Psycho-motor seizures

During a psycho-motor fit, the child's behaviour alters. There is no convulsion, no loss of consciousness. The child continues to respond to those around him, but in a limited way. There are all sorts of individual variations. The child may smell non-existent nasty smells or get a feeling of déjà vu, of 'having been here before'. Some children see things that are not there, others have violent outbursts of temper. It is uncommon for a child to experience more than one attack a day. Psycho-motor attacks are rarely seen before the age of ten, but there may have been a history of abnormal behaviour, bedwetting, nightmares or sleep-walking.

Psycho-motor attacks are sometimes known as 'temporal lobe epilepsy', because the abnormal brain activity takes place in the temporal lobe only. There may be underlying disease. Your doctor will advise about treatment.

George came from an epileptic family. His great-grandmother, his father and a brother all suffered from grand mal fits. Everything went well for him until he was seven. At this age he was not reading very satisfactorily and used to have outbursts of temper which were put down to frustration at his own under-achievement. He used to wet himself while he was angry. His IQ was tested and it was thought that he was a slow learner, but it was uniformly average (WISC-R score, 92).

By the age of nine, his temper tantrums were violent. They occurred about once every six weeks, but in between there were minor ones when it was noticed that he was forgetful. These small outbursts happened about twice a week. On assessment, his reading comprehension was a year behind, his spelling was poor and his maths not bad.

An electroencephalogram [121] showed an area of abnormal brain-cell activity and he was put on carbamazepine (which does not affect reading skills adversely). This controlled his epilepsy and his concentration so that he was able to work steadily at a slow pace. His reading and spelling kept pace as time elapsed, that is, he did not slip any further behind than when first tested. But he began to read for pleasure, and when his family left for Scotland it was felt that he was all set for take-off.

Interestingly enough, the original referral to the clinic had been made by an eye specialist, who got fed up with seeing him. The referral letter said: 'He complains of difficulty in reading and close work. He is being perpetually referred to different ophthalmologists for assessment of this. I have examined him and found that his eyes are quite normal. Could he be dyslexic?'

Focal seizures

Something happens to one part of the child's body: there's an uncontrollable twitch of a hand or foot or the corner of the mouth. The child may get funny feelings in one part only. Sometimes the movements or sensations spread to other parts of the body. An observer may see the child's eyes turning away and he may stare intently at his clenched fist. There may or may not be loss of consciousness.

This type of fit is commonly associated with some underlying local disease of the brain. Like all epilepsy, there must be proper investigation to determine the cause and therefore the right treatment.

Arnold had a perfectly normal birth, developed well and did all the right things at the right times until he got to school. His handwriting and spelling were poor, but not so bad as to excite much attention. Then suddenly, when he was eight, he had a convulsion. He was playing in his bedroom when his mother heard an odd noise and Arnold staggered into the kitchen with his face distorted. He said that his face had gone numb and then he had felt sick. He had tried to call his mother but could not. His legs would not work properly. He recovered quickly.

The electroencephalogram [121] showed epileptic activity in the mid-temporal region of the right cerebral hemisphere [56]. The clinical psychologist found that he was of average intelligence, but commented that his scores in the vocabulary and coding sub-tests of the WISC-R [68, 69] were below average. His silent reading comprehension in the GAP test [166] was at the eight years and three months level, but he made twenty-five per cent errors in the Peters 100-word spelling test for his age [173]. His handwriting and dexterity were poor. As a result of treatment, the electroencephalogram improved and the area of epileptic activity vanished. His reading improved with time but his handwriting remained poor. A year after the epilepsy was under control, he was writing 'a' and 'd' backwards, and formed '7' and '9' from below. Most letters were written in a hurried and jerky way. His family did have a Commodore microcomputer and it was suggested that he could use a word-processing program to edit written work, copying out the final draft from the VDU. As his maths was at a standstill, it was recommended that he use ready-made programs to help him overcome various mathematical stumbling-blocks of which he was aware. The local education authority was known to be prepared to advise on suitable materials for both the subject-matter and the particular machine, so his parents were asked to contact his teacher for guidance. Finally they were warned not to let the telescreen flicker while he was watching it, lest the light stimulation should cause headache or at worst another convulsion.

The electroencephalogram

121 If a paediatrician suspects that a child has epilepsy, he will ask for an electroencephalogram to confirm the diagnosis.

Brain activity is partly electrical, and it is possible to measure changes in electrical potential on the scalp, using the electroencephalogram. Round discs (the electrodes) are put on the scalp and kept in place by some sticky jelly. They are wired up to a recording machine and the child is asked to lie still and quiet while tracings of the brain's electrical output are made. No electricity passes into the child, and there are no needle pricks or anything more unpleasant than the sticky jelly. The child is encouraged to drop off to sleep and most do this. The whole process takes under an hour. The information obtained may confirm the presence of epileptic areas in the brain, or it may show to what extent the brain has matured in general. It is also used to find out how quickly the child's brain is growing. So do not jump to the conclusion that, if the doctor asks for an electroencephalogram, he suspects epilepsy; he is probably interested in the degree of development rather than the possibility of fits.

Drugs in epilepsy

122 The drugs which control epilepsy are invaluable, but if not used properly may cause problems. It is now the usual practice to monitor drug control of the disease by testing the levels of the medicine in the bloodstream. It is important to keep appointments for this monitoring, or things may get out of control.

Phenobarbitone used to be used extensively for epilepsy, but has been largely superseded; if taken for long periods it may have an effect on memory and comprehension. *Phenytoin*, now a commonly used anti-epileptic, may upset reading ability or lower general intellectual functioning, so careful control by blood-testing is always used. *Carbamazepine* now often replaces phenytoin; it seems to have a positively beneficial effect on some children's learning, though more investigations are required before this supposition is confirmed. In all cases, and whatever the medicine used, parents must stick to the dose prescribed and must not change it except under medical instruction. Withdrawing the drug suddenly 'because Johnny has not had a fit for a year' may induce a fit – stopping medication has to be done slowly and carefully. Doubling the dose because of fear that a fever or a cold may induce attacks is also wrong; it may push the blood levels up to undesirable heights. Lastly, always get a new prescription before the old one runs out and make sure that the drug dosage is reviewed at least twice a year.

Charlotte was nearly eleven when she was channelled to a special class for children whose learning disabilities were frankly medical in origin. She suffered from grand mal epilepsy, with the condition well controlled by drugs.

In class she was extremely quiet, extremely hesitant before all tasks, quite sure she could not perform even the ones she had done perfectly the week before. She needed many triggers for her memory not only to start a previously learnt routine, but also to go through with it to completion. She spoke very little, seldom volunteered information and although she was learning all the time she did it so slowly that she was, in general, about three years behind what would be expected at her age. At the start of the summer term her teachers heard that she was in hospital to have her medication adjusted. Would she return with her self-confidence and learning progress shakier still? She missed four weeks of school. The fifth Wednesday the classroom door opened, in strode Charlotte laughing and in full conversational spate, and advanced on the assembled teachers and children like a battleship with all guns blazing. In the remaining nine weeks of term she caught up by at least six months in every aspect of reading, writing, spelling and number work. Investigations showed that her drug dosage had been too high. Readjustment under strict chemical supervision produced the changes in mood and performance while still enabling her to live a fit-free life. She was able to go on to her secondary school full of self-confidence and with her competence rising daily.

Epilepsy in school

Several factors associated with epilepsy may have an impact on school performance. Psychiatric illness, a lowered intelligence, missing out on what is happening in class and the effects of drugs can all be important.

Psychiatric disorders and the poor behaviour which goes with them occur four times more often among children with epilepsy than

123

among those without it. The epileptic child shows no specific pattern of psychiatric illness or of behaviour; he acts in the same way as the other children, with the same psychiatric disorder or the same behaviour problems, but he has fits and they do not. If fits started early in life or if there is an underlying brain disorder, there may be some lowering of intelligence. Children with ideopathic (spontaneous) epilepsy generally have normal IQs, though there may be a difference between the verbal and performance scores of the WISC-R [67] There may be backwardness or even specific retardation in reading [164]. The more often the fits occur, the greater the learning disability and the worse the school performance.

Children with petit mal [120] miss out twenty or more times a day; their educational experience is shot full of holes of unconsciousness, like a tin can peppered with buckshot. As detailed in the last paragraph, some of the drugs used to control epilepsy may have an effect on reading.

Though both parents and teachers may be aware that a child suffers from epilepsy, there are some children who develop it for the first time while at school. Petit mal is by far the hardest to spot. Its late onset and the very brief duration of each attack make it almost impossible for the class teacher to see anything except a falling-off in general performance. It is a possible diagnosis which must always be borne in mind when investigating a child for dyslexia.

It is very important that a parent does not suppress information about epilepsy, even if the child is only having fits at night. There is an understandable tendency to feel that, because the attacks only occur when he is in bed, there is no need to tell anyone. The child may develop petit mal during the day, behavioural or reading problems may be puzzling the teacher, and she should know what handicaps the child has to cope with. Both the school doctor and the educational psychologist will have considerable contributions to make for the child, so do make sure that the school is informed about epilepsy if your child is unfortunate enough to have it.

There was a family history of epilepsy, but no record of Gavin ever having had a fit. His birth and childhood were uneventful, nothing medically notable happening during his first few years at school. By the time he was seven, he was not doing well in class: his compositions were poor, his grasp of simple mathematics non-existent and he was said to be inattentive, always asking what had just been said. The catch phrase 'could do better if he tried' littered his school reports. At home, he was thought to be a bit clumsy, prone to dropping things. He often wet his bed.

We found that his reading ability was about two years behind the expected level, his spelling was not bad, but his handwriting was awful. The speech therapist said that while he was carrying out tasks to instruction he twice paused and then did the task which he had just done, instead of the one she had asked him to do. She wondered if he might not have petit mal. When drawing shapes with the occupational therapist, he suddenly dropped his pencil – something children rarely do. She, too, queried the possibility of petit mal. On medical examination there was nothing to find, but an electroencephalogram [121] showed that he was having a large number of very brief seizures.

Referral to the paediatrician resulted in treatment and an overall improvement in his performance.

Epilepsy after school

Public attitudes to epilepsy are changing for the better and the chances of employment increasing for sufferers from the disease. Even so, the long-term effects may make it difficult for an epileptic to obtain rewarding employment or the qualifications necessary to satisfy his intellectual capacity.

124

Luke was first seen in the clinic when he was eighteen. He was having difficulty in coping with the reading and spelling necessary to obtain a City and Guilds qualification in a strictly practical craft. He had suffered from grand mal epilepsy since the age of six, when he had had his first attack. He had been treated with phenytoin and phenobarbitone since then. Enquiry revealed that he had had only three seizures, the last one when he was eight.

The first investigation necessary was a repeat of the electroencephalogram to confirm that he still had an area of overactivity in the parietal lobe of the right cerebral hemisphere [56]. This was indeed the case; the prolonged treatment had been justified, for without it he would probably have continued to have seizures. His I Q was estimated, using the adult form of the Wechsler test as he was too old for the WISC-R [67]. His score in the verbal I Q test was 101 and in the performance I Q 105, both within the average range. The psychologist carried out further tests and found that he had the problems with attention which often go hand-in-hand with epilepsy, but more significantly that he had a specific difficulty with spatial memory.

The speech therapist found that his language development was satisfactory. Not surprisingly, his reading comprehension age was, in the Neale test, nine years and one month, and in the GAP test, eight years and eleven months [165, 166]. His spelling was even worse.

These levels of attainment were inadequate for ordinary purposes and he was in fact illiterate.

As his work was manual and in the practice of his craft he would need very little reading or spelling, the Examining Board was asked if they would allow him to provide oral answers to oral questions in view of his disability. When they said yes, then teaching on a strictly oral basis, with tape recordings for revision, was set up and he was able to go ahead with training.

It is uncertain whether any alteration in the form of medication would have made any difference; by the time Luke was seen at the clinic there was no way of knowing. But his case does serve to underline the importance of finding out what form epilepsy takes (in this instance, right parietal overactivity) and tailoring teaching accordingly. Close cooperation between teacher, psychologist and neurologist is essential at an early stage.

Summary (120–24)
Epilepsy means having fits.
Fever convulsions in infancy are usually not due to epilepsy.
There are several different forms.
Petit mal is the hardest to spot. It develops during school years and can happen unnoticed in class.
Epilepsy can affect school performance.
The drugs taken to control epilepsy can also affect school performance, especially if not monitored properly.

The diagnosis of epilepsy is confirmed by the electroencephalogram, a non-invasive, painless procedure.

The unhappy child

An unhappy child is difficult to live with; his misery has an impact on everyone around him, especially his mother. His emotional upset may be directly associated with a physical disorder, particularly if it is one affecting brain function. What causes a learning disability may also cause an emotional disturbance.

Things may go wrong for the unhappy child at home or at school. If he can just about cope, then he will react. If he cannot cope, he may develop a physical disorder in much the same way as a tense businessman gets ulcers. Most commonly several factors combine to create the final situation, so that parents find it difficult to know why their child should be naughty, attention-seeking, restless at night and clumsy, why he should suffer head- and stomach-aches and do badly at school.

It is easy for parents to feel guilty and to blame themselves for all their child's troubles and poor behaviour. 'What did we do wrong?' It is easy to blame one's spouse or hug the blame to oneself. It is difficult to ask for help if you feel that it's all your own fault. It can be a relief for parents to learn that they are faced with a physical reason for their child's dyslexia, but, by the same token, it is all too easy to take refuge behind some sort of medical label. The easiest thing is to be an author and hand out general advice; the most difficult thing is to be a parent and know which course to follow.

If you are aware that your child needs help, it is useful to consider that his problems may arise from one or more of the following causes:

- there may be a medical reason;
- he may be fit, but he may be reflecting family or school disturbances;
- he may be in the wrong school.

Identifying the sources of stress make it easier to decide what to do to help him.

Symptoms which must not be ignored

Children with learning disabilities may complain of something or have symptoms which seem to be ploys for not having to go to school, but which must not be dismissed lightly. The commonest are stomach-aches and headaches.

125

126

Stomach-ache

Pain in the tummy which comes on in the morning and is so bad that the child cannot get up or cannot walk properly must always provoke a parental response. Quite rightly, the first reaction is to take him to the doctor to see if it is appendicitis or some other physical disease. If the doctor is not sure, he may recommend a short stay in hospital for observation. If the outcome is favourable and there is no physical disease, it is easy to feel that the child is putting it on just to get out of going to school. Intestinal colic from tension or emotional upset is very uncomfortable. Just think of the sudden guts-ache you got when that motorbike nearly hit you, or you were near an explosion. Do not dismiss his belly-ache as a con trick. If the cause is emotional, this needs sorting out just as the inflamed appendix needs taking out. The child is often the first to recognize his own inadequacies, and the stomach-ache may be the first hint of a learning disability. So if your doctor assures you that the cause is not physical, get together with the teacher to see if you can identify the underlying problem.

Recurrent headaches

Of course, if your child is about to develop mumps or go down with flu, he will get a headache as his fever rises. What must be of concern to you is the recurring headache. There are many different causes for this. A simple checklist may underline the need to seek medical advice:

1. Chronic infections of the sinuses or the throat may produce persistent headaches, as may a generalized infection such as glandular fever.

2. Poor vision, where glasses are needed and perhaps prescribed but not worn, may result in headache.

3. If a parent suffers from migraine, the child may do so too (do not forget that there is an abdominal form of this).

4. He may be accustomed to headaches in the household and his ache-threshold may be low, so that slight discomforts swell to imitate the parental migraine.

5. Early-morning epilepsy, barely noticed at that time in the day, produces post-convulsion headaches, often with a wet bed.

6. In the older age groups, drug or alcohol abuse may first become obvious because of the hangover.

7. There are rare and serious conditions which raise the tension inside the skull.

All these causes may be confused with an anxiety headache. So get your doctor to check, before you dismiss his symptom as being 'psychological' or a try-on. If there is nothing physically wrong, then – as with stomach-aches – get together with the teacher to see if you can find out what is bothering your child.

Wetting and soiling

Wetting and soiling by the schoolchild isolate him from his peer group despite the best efforts of teachers and parents. Constipation with overflow soiling may be associated with the sequencing problems of dyslexia. The symptoms require investigation to exclude disease and should not be regarded as stress induced until other possible causes have been excluded.

Sources of stress

Not only does the learning-disabled child suffer from behavioural problems because of his physical condition but he may be affected by stressful situations, as other children are.

127

Lack of mothering, due either to unavoidable absence because of maternal physical illness, or withdrawal because of depressive disease, may retard his development in all spheres. If the mother becomes ill and unable to tend her child, then a knowledgeable substitute must be found, preferably one the child knows. That is what grannies are for. Death, whether of a parent, grandparent, brother, sister, friend or even a pet, may produce anxiety and feelings of guilt. A child may become fearful lest other members of the family should die too. Parental separation or divorce may be akin to death for a child. He may feel responsible in some way. Whatever the rights and wrongs of the break-up of a marriage, the child must be considered and advice sought for his emotional wellbeing. The lawyers will look after the money matters, but a child psychiatrist may be able to advise on emotional questions. Re-marriage, too, can be stressful for him; coping with stepfather and stepbrothers or sisters is not easy. Bullying, sexual abuse, fear of street violence are all too common causes of stress. One-parent families face particular problems. The lack of a father may make a child try to become the man about the house and he may adopt an unusually aggressive attitude at school.

Poverty can have a dire effect on the family and sometimes comes after a death or a divorce. The mother may have such a struggle to feed, clothe and keep her children warm that she has no time for anything else. There may be little time for language development and no play time. Discipline may become inconsistent when she is worn-out and tired. Normal adventurous behaviour on the part of the child may be rewarded by inappropriate punishment. The family may mistrust authority. Their very physical existence may depend on circumventing the law. Policemen and teachers may be seen as hostile, their only purpose being the curtailing of the family's economic success. Where existence is hand to mouth, the Artful Dodger is bred.

Under any of these adverse circumstances, the learning-disabled child is at a double disadvantage.

Some stress effects

128

There is a graduated scale of reactions to stress which ranges from beneficial stimulation through worry to anxiety or depression and, rarely, to complete nervous breakdown. The nature of a particular child colours his reactions. Ill-health will make him vulnerable. The severity of an adverse reaction is dependent on the persistence and degree of the stress.

In a fit child there may be a reversion to an earlier stage of development, 'playing baby', with demands for attention, stomach-aches or headaches, temper tantrums and tears too often. Take away the stress and the reactions subside. Jenny's story illustrates this.

Jenny was a twelve-year-old girl. There was nothing of significance in her medical history. Her family were secure and successful. The father and mother were ambitious for their children, had read all the best books on child development, were eager to help and fearful of being too pushy.

After a successful time at her junior school, where she always got full marks for spelling, she went to a former grammar school turned comprehensive, 'the best school in the district'. By the time she had been there for half a term, she was coming home exhausted and irritable. She needed a lot of help with her homework. She burst into tears easily. Each morning before starting out for school she developed a stomach-ache. After a couple of trips to the family doctor to make sure that she had not got appendicitis, this was put down to nerves. Her school reported that she worked hard and that she was still good at spelling. Her essays and compositions were poor. She found maths difficult. Both her maths and English teachers said that she was inattentive. The art and physical education teachers praised her work and remarked that she concentrated well and was a great trier. Her parents paid for extra help with the maths and English, but with no beneficial results. 'Was she dyslexic?' they asked.

When she came to the clinic, nothing abnormal was found on medical examination. Her I Q, using the W I S C - R test [67], was in the average range – verbal I Q, 95; performance I Q, 92; full scale I Q, 94. On seeing this, her form mistress remarked, 'That's very low.'

She was in an academic environment above her capabilities. She was moved to a school with a truly comprehensive view of education. Her stress symptoms have gone and she has never looked back.

It is rare to encounter simple causes and simple solutions. The case of Jenny is an exception rather than a commonplace one. More often there are multiple causes, some of which it may be impossible to eliminate. A child who can just about cope with a stress may develop a variety of symptoms which, if allowed to become permanent, may severely handicap his day-to-day living. For example, all children go through periods of adherence to ritual, observing meaningless taboos with unswerving determination: 'Always spit when you see a black cat', 'Don't walk on the lines in the pavement.'

If the whole family is perfectionist, the child may become obsessed with such rituals. Some may have a purposeful basis. All the fat is cut off the food, hand-washing becomes excessive. Sacrifices are made to the demon of anxiety. As well as 'I must do', 'I must *not* do' may become prominent. School performance suffers in a general way, though there is usually no specific falling-off in reading or spelling attainment. But further advances are slowed down. If testing is carried out by an assessment team, the visual and auditory short-term memories [73] are found to be poor and concentration to be lacking. This is not surprising; anxiety makes all of us forget things.

Quite severe, almost hysterical, symptoms may become manifest and general medical conditions – seemingly unrelated to learning disabilities – may become exaggerated. The allergic child [115] becomes more so; eczema [47] flares; he wheezes, or his nose becomes stuffy. Bedwetting may become a problem. Most children are dry by the time they are three, but some persist in wetting or become dry and then start wetting again. The causes may be psychological (due to stress or an anticipated threat), neurological (nocturnal epilepsy [120], for example), or local (perhaps because of bladder or vulval irritation). Whatever the cause the child will need help, so if your boy or girl persists in bedwetting after the age of five, seek medical advice.

Helping with stress

129

Whatever one's fears of psychiatrists and psychologists, they can really help the child under stress. They identify the causes of the problem so that these may be relieved. They can help to unravel the effects of stress and prevent symptoms becoming permanent. Do not shy away from seeking such assistance. Go first to your family doctor or the school medical officer – these generalists will make sure there is no physical condition underlying the psychiatric disturbance.

If you are advised to do so by your family physician, put yourself and your child in the hands of the professionals and pay heed to what they say. Do not forget that they may see the child as their patient first and foremost, and that, like all doctors, they may respect his confidences. This may lead to a seeming reluctance on their part to discuss what your child has said to them. Respect this attitude – they may well do the same in reverse and treat as confidential your own view of your child.

Mark was eight years old. He was doing badly at school. His father and mother had separated when he was two and had legally divorced three years later. He was the younger of two children, his sister being eleven. His birth had been traumatic. Just before his arrival, his mother had suffered a brisk rise in blood pressure. At birth, he weighed 6 lbs 2 oz, the cord was wound twice round his neck and he was 'a bit blue'. He was difficult to feed at first and was a restless, irritable baby. However, he walked and talked at normal times, though his mother felt that he was always a bit clumsy.

After the divorce, his mother was not very well-off and had to go out to work. So Mark went to a day-nursery; his mother used to put him in at 8.30 each morning and pick him up again at 5.30, except at weekends,when he stayed at home with her. He had suffered from eczema as an infant and when seen in the clinic this was still obvious on his hands and arms. He had settled into his infants school quite well but had difficulty in learning to read. By the time he was six and a half, his teacher was complaining that his attention was poor and that he was disruptive in class.

At home, he easily lost his temper, fought with his sister at the slightest provocation and was possessive of his mother. If crossed, he would go into his room, lock the door and batter his toys about. At one time he stole from his mother's purse and was suspected of stealing at school.

On clinical examination, he was an itchy, twitchy boy, but the male doctor found him easy to get on with. He was a bit clumsy and uncoordinated, though not to an extent that indicated any positive neurological disease. The doctor recorded on his notes that he had 'soft' neurological signs [136]. The speech therapist found that his language development showed an overall limitation. She remarked on his poor short-term memory both for what he heard and for the order in which he saw shapes [73]. His IQ was in the average range. The remedial teacher found that his literary skills were below the expected levels for his age and intelligence.

What could be done for him? Everyone claimed him for their own. The psychologist saw him as a stress-related case of poor behaviour, the doctor as a case of minimal brain dysfunction [136], the speech therapist as a child whose language needed enriching, the teacher as a child in need of remedial help.

None of the specialists did him much good until the mother solved the problem herself. She remarried. The stepfather was a warm, easy-going man who accepted his stepson, warts and all. The financial status of the family improved.

The speech therapist gave good advice about improving his short-term memory [73]; the remedial teacher bumped up his reading age to a level acceptable to him and his school. When last heard of at the age of ten and a half, Mark and his stepfather were going off each weekend fishing. He wanted to be like his stepfather when he grew up. Everyone felt self-congratulatory at first, but on reflection we all knew that it was the new marriage, plus the stepfather's painstaking efforts with Mark, which had really solved his problems.

Depressive disease

If a child breaks a favourite toy, he is miserable. If he cannot go on a long-anticipated trip, he is unhappy. If he is ill, he is first cross and then

130

wretched. When he gets a new toy or gets better, he is happy once more.

Unhappiness is not depression.

Commonly, depression is a word implying a passing phase of misery or irritation. Circumstances change and so do our moods. Doctors mean something quite different when they talk about depressive disease. To them, this is a medical condition which has an inevitable and sometimes catastrophic effect on a child's performance at school. After partial hearing loss [27, 31, 32], it is the commonest cause of learning disabilities seen in the clinic. Depressive disease in a child is characterized by *persistent* misery; there are very few breaks in the clouds. The child sleeps badly, sometimes waking early. Breakfast-time is awful, with sullenness, bad temper, school refusal, stomach-aches. By the evening things are a bit better, though unhappiness persists. At home he fluctuates between aggressiveness and possessiveness. At school he is isolated, without friends. He is inattentive in class, never finishing work, never apparently trying. Reading and spelling will be stuck at the level of attainment when the disease first started. This means that if he comes to school with the condition, he will never learn anything.

There are some peculiar features to the disease. Children with depressive disease draw themselves in profile and they may rotate letters on their axes, 'b' for 'd', 'n' for 'u'. It is normal for a child to do this up to the age of eight, but depressives will do it when older. The rotations come and go with the severity of the disease. The sudden appearance of rotations in the writing of an older boy should always be regarded with some suspicion. They do not constitute a diagnosis of depressive disease, only a hint that it may be there. Most of all, children with the disease have difficulty in organizing their thoughts and sometimes cannot manage even such a simple task as spelling a two-syllable word. They draw a straight line instead. It is not that they don't try, but that they can't.

Depressive disease is frequently a reaction to a combination of physical and emotional trauma. A happy child may get into bed with flu. His best friend, Hammy the hamster, dies. When, apparently better, the child returns to school without a fever or a hamster, he is persistently miserable and depressed.

Treatment must be at the discretion of the family doctor and, if need be, the child psychiatrist as well. It is usually twofold. Anti-depressive medicines alleviate the condition and give the body time to work its own cure, while the child psychiatrist supplies support, perhaps over many sessions, for the child.

Until the disease is better, it is difficult for the child to absorb new ideas or concepts. The anti-depressants may fool you into thinking that, because his mood is lighter, the disease is at an end. If you make this assumption, both you and the teacher will be disappointed.

Until he has been off the pills for at least three months and the depression has truly gone, do not expect his school performance to return to normal. Beware, too, of relapses following further traumas.

Richard was an only child. There was no family history of psychiatric disorders. His mother's pregnancy had been normal and so was the delivery. He weighed 7 lbs 3 oz at birth. He was a happy, active baby. He was dry at the age of four, though he reverted to bedwetting after seeing a horror film when he was five. (He had been allowed to sit up to see it on TV.)

When he got to school, he had difficulty in making friends. By the time he was nine, he was doing very badly in class, finding spelling especially difficult. He put the letters in any order in words and reversed numerals. He mixed up words when speaking. His IQ was average: WISC-R verbal IQ, 95; performance IQ, 99; full scale, 96 [68, 69, 70]. He was diagnosed as 'dyslexic'.

When seen in the clinic at the age of ten and a half, he was clumsy. His language had developed normally, though his listening skills had not. His Neale oral reading comprehension test [165] was at the level of seven years and nine months. His silent reading comprehension, measured by the GAP test [166] was at the level of nine years. His spelling was at the level of eight years and four months.

He presented a picture of misery; he burst into tears for no apparent reason and sat slumped in a chair with no obvious interest in things around him. The child psychiatrist confirmed a diagnosis of depressive disease and started him on anti-depressant medication. Five months later his reading scores had jumped by eight months; he was happier. Treatment continued for several months. When last heard of, his depression had been left behind and at the age of seventeen he had four O-levels and was working on some more, and one A-level.

Depressive disease is not the prerogative of boys. Cherry was born normally, but at the age of four she witnessed a road accident, when the child next door was badly injured. She began to stutter and her language development became delayed. At this time her hearing was checked and found to be normal; her I Q was estimated and shown to be average.

When seen in the clinic at the age of ten, she was doing badly at school, she had few friends and she slept badly, waking very early. Going to school involved a physical fight between her and her mother, who had to drag her along. Her Neale oral reading scores [165] were: for speed, six years and six months; for accuracy, seven years; and for comprehension, six years and six months. Her spelling age in the Schonell test [173] was at the level of five years and five months.

The child psychiatrist considered that she had been suffering from depressive disease since the traumatic experience. She attended group therapy, but it was two years before she began to talk about the accident. About the third year, she began to pick up. She slept well and volunteered that she had happy dreams; she began to make friends. However, her scholastic performance remained static for about three and a half years. Eventually she got O-levels in art, biology and geography and attempted A-levels in art and geography. Spelling remained a problem and English language O-level eluded her. In order that some age allowance should be made for her, the Examining Board was sent the results of the adult form of the Wechsler Intelligence Scale which showed that she had an average verbal intelligence and a superior performance intelligence: the medical aspect of her spelling disability was emphasized.

Summary (127–30)
Stress can be good for you, except in excess.
A child under too much stress behaves badly and is unhappy.
Stress can cause stomach-aches or headaches.
Stress can cause clumsiness.
Stress can cause learning difficulties.
Learning disabilities can cause stress.
Anxiety results when a child cannot cope with stress.

Depressive disease may follow apparently slight stress.

Depressive disease is characterized by persistent misery and inefficient thought.

Depressive disease and anxiety require medical treatment.

Chapter Eleven
The Dyslexias

131

Dyslexia and acquired dyslexia

The prefix 'dys-' is used by the medical profession to indicate an abnormal function of some sort. Thus, 'dys-pepsia' means poor digestion; 'dys-entery' means inflamed bowels with diarrhoea; 'dys-lexia' means impairment of the ability to read, and nothing more. The troubles start when dyslexia becomes festooned with adjectives. Fuller meanings are implied and explanations have to follow.

When a medical term leaves the medical dictionary and becomes part of common speech, there is always confusion because what the doctors understood when they first defined the term changes and broadens in its meaning. For example, to doctors 'influenza' is a disease caused by a specific group of viruses, while to most of us it means any cold or fever occurring during the winter, severe enough to give us a day or two off work.

This has happened to dyslexia, which now has many different meanings, depending on the qualifying adjectives attached to it. There are two main categories, acquired and developmental.

Acquired dyslexia refers to the loss of a reading skill already fully developed.

Knowledge of the reading process, of what happens when we read and how we read, has been gleaned from the study of adults known to be brain damaged. The types of difficulties which such patients experience when trying to read have been related to the areas of their brains known to be damaged. Destruction of one small part of the brain from, say, a stroke or a gunshot wound is associated with one type of reading difficulty, whilst destruction of another area in a different patient is associated with a totally different sort of dyslexia. Acquired dyslexia may be divided into five forms 'surface', 'visual', 'deep', 'phonological' and 'direct'.

Surface dyslexics read silently by ear and recognize words by sounds and not by the picture each word makes on paper. This technique does not allow for the vagaries of English spelling, for example 'where' and 'wear'. Such patients fail to understand what they are reading because the meaning of the pronounced word may be quite different from that of the written one.

Visual dyslexics confuse words in which the general configuration of letters is similar. They may read 'hay' as 'lip', or 'punt' as 'gash' because the loops and uprights make similar patterns. However, they can spell out the individual letters in a word, but not put them together correctly. Some may slowly spell out each letter of a word, trying, often unsuccessfully, to put them together in order to recognize the whole.

Deep dyslexics are not able to use phonics; they cannot convert what they see on the page into the known sounds of the letters or combinations of letters. They look at a word and will probably read out one of equivalent meaning – we know a patient who read 'city' as 'Liverpool'. Deep dyslexics can usually read words referring to familiar things like 'table' or 'bed', but have difficulty with the meaning of abstract words.

Phonological dyslexics do not have the deep dyslexic's problem with the meaning of abstract words, but do have difficulty coping with the sounds of syllables or individual letters.

Direct dyslexics can read fluently, but do not understand what they have read. When they read aloud, it sounds good but that is all; their comprehension is lacking.

By combining the information obtained from patients with acquired dyslexia together with studies of the way competent adults read, it is possible to design different models of the reading process. Such a model may resemble a child's board game, where arrows point to the first goal from which other arrows lead to the next one, each goal having a different title. A really good model-maker will create at least eight such goals with different routes between them. The different types of acquired dyslexia can be related to disturbances in the appropriate goal. The result of such disturbances is a failure to make sense of the text that has been read. It is important to appreciate that any model is but a suggestion of the original, and that model-makers may be tempted to use only information which makes their model comprehensible; such models are 'guestimates' of what happens to enable us to read. None of them is sacrosanct and each is liable to suffer change as the result of increasing scientific knowledge.

Developmental dyslexia and specific developmental dyslexia
Developmental dyslexia is the failure of the reading ability of a child to develop normally due to the effects of some illness or trauma.

132

Although there is a superficial resemblance between the patterns of acquired dyslexia and those seen in developmental dyslexia, it is misleading to extrapolate from the adult's picture to the child's. The adult has grown up normally and is damaged with obvious effect. The child is still growing; development has yet to be completed; the effects of a disease on reading development depend not only on the nature of the disease but also on the stage of development at which it strikes. For example, the effects of deafness on the development of a child's language (and therefore on his reading ability later) vary with the age at which the child becomes deaf. The similarity between the acquired and developmental dyslexias is that the difficulty with reading is, for both, a symptom, that is, the result of a disease.

Specific developmental dyslexia was mentioned very briefly at the beginning of the book [2]. It is now time to consider the term in greater detail. There are three phrases which cover roughly the same field of learning disabilities:

1. Specific developmental dyslexia describes what a child cannot do – that is, read, write or spell – as well as everyone thinks he should.

2. Attention deficit disorder describes what a child unfortunately does do, namely behaves in a way that irritates or angers adults.

3. Minimal brain dysfunction, a vague medical term, tries to account for both the specific developmental dyslexia and the attention deficit disorder.

Specific developmental dyslexia has been defined by the World Federation of Neurology as 'a disorder manifested by difficulty in learning to read despite conventional instruction, adequate intelligence and socio-cultural opportunity. It is dependent upon fundamental cognitive disabilities which are frequently of constitutional origin.' The absence of reference to spelling is surprising.

Since that original definition was made, other features have been ascribed to the condition. These are: discrepancies between spelling performance and intellectual capacity, confusion of 'b' with 'd', difficulty in distinguishing right from left [79], difficulty in repeating polysyllabic words or digits in reverse order, difficulty in learning the times tables, clumsiness [81], late walking [76] and late talking [93, 94]. Latterly the phrase 'specific developmental dyslexia' has been narrowed to just 'dyslexia'. This causes much confusion, not least because enthusiasts publish very long lists of 'symptoms of dyslexia' and leave it simply at a list. There is no attempt to explain links between particular symptoms and possible causes. This turns dyslexia into a condition rather than a symptom. It also ignores the rich potential for understanding and amelioration implied by the view that dyslexia is just one feature of a wide range of disabilities present in the community at large.

Children who are specifically retarded in their reading can be defined quite precisely on a statistical basis which takes into account their age and intelligence as determined by an IQ test [67]. If there is no demonstrable reason for their retardation, then and only then may they be said to be suffering from 'specific developmental dyslexia'. In short, it is a diagnosis by exclusion.

The symptoms additional to reading retardation are shared by other conditions, in much the same way as spots and fever go with both measles and German measles. Differences between spelling performance and intellectual capacity may occur with delayed language development [93, 94] or poor listening skills [98], both of which are consequent on middle-ear disease [31]. Clumsiness [81] and difficulty with polysyllabic words may be associated with neurological disorder [91], while rotations of 'b' and 'd' may occur with depressive disease [130]. One school of thought suggests that alterations in male hormone levels in the foetus are related to learning difficulties in left-handed people. If this hypothesis is proved right it will further reduce the number of specific – that is, cause unknown – dyslexics. Before these finer distinctions were made, specific developmental dyslexia covered too wide a field to serve much purpose. Three sub-divisions, 'visual', 'auditory' and 'mixed', were described, each covering a particular pattern of difficulty in learning to read.

Visual specific developmental dyslexics cannot easily recognize words just by looking at them – they are word-blind – but are strong on phonics and respond to teaching using phonic materials. Their right/left cerebral hemisphere balance seems tilted to the left [57].

Auditory specific developmental dyslexics are the reverse. They have no problem remembering and reading by sight, but do not respond to a phonic approach. The hemisphere balance seems to tilt to the right.

The mixed category shows characteristics of both the other two types. They have the worst of both worlds, but usually in milder form. These descriptions, however precise, give no indication of the cause of the dyslexia. If it is not known why a child should be dyslexic, then both the prognosis and treatment cannot be determined with any accuracy. Faced with a dyslexic pupil, the teacher has to decide whether to attempt to improve a weakness or to make the most of the child's strengths. An accurate diagnosis would tell her whether the weakness she observed was there to stay or was only temporary and could be strengthened by appropriate remedial teaching. At best, categorizing a child as being a visual or auditory dyslexic does not tell the teacher enough for her to plan her teaching strategies. She will be driven back on empirical methods and day-to-day experimentation. 'I'll try this and if it doesn't work I'll try that.'

A book about dyslexia that includes descriptions of cases seen must include at least one description of a child suffering from it. Easy, you would think, when the authors had been working in the field for years. Not a bit of it. While for all the other slots cases came to mind after at most the briefest discussion, the 'SDD child' had us stumped. Of whom could we honestly say that in our professional judgement SDD pure and simple was the cause of the trouble? Was there a child for whom SDD was the major cause of the trouble? The substantial cause of the trouble? The deadline approached and passed, and no obvious case came to mind.

> *Summary (131–2)*
> *Dyslexia has two meanings:*
> *a. the strictly scientific one, that of impairment of reading ability.*
> *b. the common usage one that my child is not learning to read as well as he should.*
> *Acquired Dyslexia is the failure of reading ability in a competent adult as the result of disease. There are several patterns.*
> *Developmental Dyslexia is the failure of a child to acquire reading normally due to disease or trauma. Specific Developmental Dyslexia, sometimes shortened to Dyslexia, is the failure of a child to acquire reading normally for no recognizable cause.*

Attention deficit disorder

133 Attention deficit disorder includes, as a description, children who have some degree of inattention, are somewhat impulsive and usually over-active, their overall behaviour being unacceptable to adults.

You must bear in mind that children may be restless for different reasons:

- children with distinct neurological problems may be restless or fearless;
- the partially deaf child may have difficulty in concentrating or understanding what is asked of him;

- an anxious child may be scared that his home life is about to disintegrate or that his parents may vanish;
- threadworms irritate the anus and may make a child wriggle;
- the specially gifted child, bored to tears and therefore inattentive, may appear overactive.

All these possibilities will be treated at length, as they deserve, but one must be cleared out of the way now: hyperkinesis. The term is almost a synonym for attention deficit disorder. It is worth comparing these two conditions in detail.

Hyperkinesis

134

What does the word mean? 'Hyper' means 'over much' and 'kinesis' means 'motion'; strictly the word implies overmuch bodily movement, with little suggestion of the bluebottle turn of mind which many of these children exhibit. In common parlance, the words 'hyperkinesis', 'hyperactivity' and 'overactivity' have all come to mean the same thing. To include the impulsiveness and mental restlessness, the new term 'attention deficit disorder' is now used.

Unfortunately, the term 'hyperkinesis' changes meaning when it crosses the Atlantic, having a broader meaning and encompassing more children in the United States than it does in Great Britain. There are thought to be about 4 per cent of children in the USA with attention deficit disorder, while only about 0.01 per cent of children in Great Britain are hyperactive. This difference is not due to any medical or environmental factors but rather to different use of similar terms. In the States, the term is used of children who may be inattentive, impulsive, and often – but not always – overactive. In addition, they usually have learning problems, may be rather negative, have a quick temper and be inclined to bully. The onset of these symptoms is usually before the age of three and always before seven. The condition must last for six months or more. Children with frank psychiatric illness, such as depressive disease, are excluded, as are those who are mentally retarded. In Great Britain, the term is confined to those children who are so markedly overactive that they never rest and are virtually unteachable, unless treated.

So what does the unfortunate parent see? It is one of the features of the hyperkinetic child, whichever definition is used, that he behaves in an exemplary fashion in the doctor's office and leaves his parent saying, 'If only you could see him at home, doctor.' So both the doctor in Cambridge, Massachusetts, and the doctor in Cambridge, East Anglia, will need information from the parents before he can arrive at a classification. The mother needs to know the difference between a child's normal boisterous activity and abnormal overactivity.

You can expect your two-year-old to be into everything. Having tasted the fun of discovery, he reaches up for things, pulls electric plugs out of their sockets if he can, will get at the hot shiny kettle, pushes little cars about the floor and up your legs, and clutches at dolls and piles of bricks indiscriminately. He will grab things from another toddler and will hang on for dear life to the favourite item of the moment. Try to take it away and you will meet real resistance. He should not be still until he drops off to sleep, flopped out and happy. Is this hyperkinesis? Certainly not; it's normal, it's what you did at the same age – and what a fun age it is, though be on your guard as your infant Hercules gives the flex an exploratory tug. It is the puppy stage, puddles and all.

The two-year-old hyperkinetic child is an exaggeration. He scarcely slept in his earlier months and now he does not seem to sleep at all. The flat-out, settled-down moments when you can put your feet up, or say: 'Sssh – he's asleep, but it doesn't matter, nothing will wake him', just never come. He gives you no peace, but is not apparently affected, though the same cannot be said for you.

By three, most children will be sharing things with friends and will be playing with them rather than on their own. Though he asks endless questions, he will also talk to himself, often about what he is doing at the time. He is fond and likes to help you.

The hyperkinetic child is always on the go, restless and unable to sit still. He finds it difficult to join in play with other children and, when he does, is so easily distracted from what he should be doing that he upsets the party. He never stays with one game or activity for any time at all. If you try to get him to join in and help, you will find that he has gone before you have finished talking.

By four, children should be cheeky and determined to do what they want. They need their friends and they fluctuate between being bossy and being cooperative. Dressing-up takes place regularly and hide-outs are built in the garden. They know the justice of taking turns, and they get upset if a friend is hurt and cries.

The hyperkinetic child is a menace to himself at this age. He rushes into dangerous situations without thinking and traffic can be a real problem. You dare not let him out of your sight. It is not easy to keep up with him because he is so active and runs about or climbs heedlessly. Worse, he never rests, so you dare not either. He never plays with other children, or if he does he spoils it all by never playing the part allotted to him.

It was bad enough at four; it's worse at five. Five-year-olds are normally sensible, well-controlled and cautious. Games are thought out beforehand and carried right through to the end. Friends are important and fair play to the fore. Young brothers or sisters are looked after and, if need be, defended.

The hyperkinetic child is still on the go at five, still impulsive, still a danger to himself, much more so now there's more of him and he's more mobile. You, of course, are still worn out.

A normal form of hyperactivity

135

In contrast to the child who is restless in class because he cannot meet the demands made on him, there is the child who is spectacularly inattentive because he is far brighter than the average. Not that parents and teachers are at first aware of this. All they know is that the child's everyday behaviour has driven them to exhaustion or screaming or both.

In class the child will perform solo tasks rapidly and well, especially new ones. With familiarity, performance may become careless, while remaining very quick. So with a lovely lot of free time he will busy himself inventing games, trying out new activities or reorganizing familiar ones, often accompanying himself with a voluble and well-expressed running commentary. He will not stay still except while absorbed in some sedentary task and he will not pay attention to the teacher for what she considers to be the necessary minimum. He will be physically and mentally on the move, seeming never to stop for breath. If he is bossy, group tasks may find him rejected by his peers, giving him more opportunities to entertain himself. If rejected too often, he may withdraw and become absorbed in a satisfying world of his own, isolated from his age group, playing with older children. If he is also large, this works well.

At home, with more adult interaction, he should theoretically be easier to live with. That is seldom the case, at least while he is young. For a start the chances are that he will sleep very little and demand entertainment or the company of some member of the family during all his waking hours. These are the children, who, as babies, dismantle their cots or prams, open up light plugs, and so on. Tired parents fill their cots with toys in the hope of getting an extra half hour of sleep. It doesn't work, for the irregular drop-drop of bricks – which are greatly enjoyed – sliding off the blankets is insistently rousing. When older, they often start large collections, organize and reorganize them and invade all the corners of the home with them. They will play elaborate pretend games, make all the props and try to involve the entire family in them. They are always ready for the next, more interesting activity, and very very cross, however briefly, if frustrated.

It is obviously desirable to find out from a psychologist, using formal testing, how bright such a child actually is. If the figures are at or beyond a given magic threshold, it will be possible to join an organization like the National Association for Gifted Children, which will provide weekend entertainment for the child and advice to parents on how to manage him. But even without a psychologist, there are several things parents can do to make their own and the child's life easier:

1. Teach him to read at the earliest opportunity; keep him supplied with books and give him a bedside light.

2. If you can, give him a room of his own where he can get up and play as early or as late as it suits him.

3. Keep his mind fed and stretched, but without allowing him to withdraw. So encourage hobbies, with their related clubs; outings with the family or friends or school or club; learning to play a musical instrument in a group with a teacher; using a microcomputer. Always explain what he is doing and why – adult conversation all along the line, with expression as full, accurate and correct (and, when he is older, stylistically appropriate) as possible. See how far school can provide 'enrichment' programmes; can he start extra subjects, take exams early? How about some absorbing sport? This, too, feeds the imagination and reminds him of his dependence on the ninety-five per cent less bright than himself. But overall, keep him stretched and insist on the highest standards.

Minimal brain dysfunction

136 Minimal brain dysfunction, sometimes called minimal cerebral dysfunction or MBD for short, seems to be a precise definition of a medical condition. But it does not stand up very well to scientific analysis. It turns out to be like an after-dinner speech: concise, plausible, but not very informative. In essence, it implies that the brain is not working as well as it should; the very word 'minimal' means 'do not worry too much, it is only a mild sort of problem'.

The idea of MBD has been part of the neurological contribution to the puzzle of learning disabilities. It is the medical, or biological, factor in contrast to psychological and behavioural ones.

It was formulated as a concept when it was thought that children who suffered from brain infections or injuries developed hyperactivity, poor behaviour and learning problems. This was followed by the proposal that damage resulting from a stormy birth produced a similar picture, most obvious when the child went to school. There was thought to be a spectrum of ill-effects arising from birth trauma which ranged from death, through cerebral palsy to specific dyslexia to normality. Looking at cerebral-palsied children, doctors could find positive signs of disease in the nervous system, perceptual difficulties, clumsiness, purposeless movements, and epilepsy sometimes with abnormal electro-encephalograms and learning disabilities. Further along the spectrum, doctors could find the same sort of learning disabilities, perceptuo-motor deficits, clumsiness, overactivity, poor behaviour and poor concen- tration, abnormal electroencephalograms and what are termed 'soft' neurological signs. These are slightly abnormal signs which the doctor finds when he probes and prods his patient. For example, there may be difficulty in balancing, in touching the thumbs with the fingers in quick succession, and in twisting the wrists at speed. There are a host of these 'soft' signs. They do not identify positively the site of any damage in the nervous system. It is sometimes difficult to be certain whether they indicate a delay in development or whether they point to some underlying disease.

At various times, opinions have fluctuated on the question of whether MBD is a permanent state of affairs extending into adult life (that is, it is due to damage), or whether it is just a hiccup in normal development, any learning difficulties being secondary. Over the years, the abnormalities which are associated with MBD have been extended and now cover a wide field. Hyperkinesis, clumsiness due to lack of awareness of body position, poor perception, language delays, bad behaviour, learning disabilities and 'soft' signs are all included. Altogether, there are too many abnormalities to make the clinical picture of MBD clear-cut. It can be used only after a specialist medical examination.

It has also become apparent that not all the children who have suffered birth trauma develop learning disabilities later, so the idea that perinatal problems necessarily cause brain damage or dysfunction has given way to the realization that an increased *risk* of trouble results, rather than a certainty of it.

There remain two jokers in the pack of information. First, learning disabilities are known to run in families, and second, more boys than girls are affected. The possibility that there might be some alteration in brain chemistry, of genetic origin, has to be considered.

The current thinking is that there is no single cause for the medley of signs, symptoms and learning disabilities covered by the wide umbrellas of MBD, attention deficit disorder and specific developmental dyslexia. A number of events, diseases or poisons may affect the child's brain. In some cases, the clinical picture and the effects are known, in others there is only a suspicion that they are harmful and related to learning disabilities. What is not clear is the relation between various untoward events and the different types of learning disabilities which are known to exist. If a mother suffers from disease A when she is X number of months pregnant, will her baby develop a specific type of learning disability later? Does disease A link only with spelling problems of a certain sort? Such questions do not yet have answers.

Therapies

137

Historically, specific developmental dyslexia was regarded as an entity – a syndrome – a positively identifiable condition which must therefore have a cause. With increasing knowledge, this approach has lost favour and there has been a swing from the original conception of it as an illness to its being a symptom, which may result from many different causes. Before the swing got under way, several theories were put forward to account for the occurrence of specific developmental dyslexia; as a consequence of these, therapies were formulated in the expectation of making the learning disability better.

The most popular explanation was that it was due to a deficiency in visual processing and memory associated with minimal brain dysfunction. Programmes were devised to improve visual perception with the intention of secondarily improving the dyslexia.

A theory postulating an intersensory deficit was also popular. It associated reading disabilities with difficulty in integrating all the information coming into the brain from the sensory systems. 'Integrating' means using relevant and discarding irrelevant information from the eyes, ears, nose, skin and sense-of-position organs and passing that information from one side of the brain to the other.

From this last theory have arisen a number of therapeutic programmes designed to improve a child's sensory integration. The therapist subjects the child to all kinds of enjoyable activities involving movement, stimulation by touch and stimulation of the semi-circular canal system [25]. The intervention aims to enhance integration of the sensory systems. From the child's point of view, he has a jolly time being rubbed with a dry cloth, brushed if he enjoys that, spun about in a net, allowed to roll all over the place on a large ball or encouraged to pull himself around on a skateboard. He gains experience of his own self, of the world about him, of gravity and of movement.

There is little really convincing evidence that such a programme has a direct effect on reading or other learning disabilities. However, stimulation of and interaction with the pre-school child by a communicating, friendly adult does a great deal to improve a child's self-confidence, language and perception of himself and space. This is definitely beneficial, rather than therapeutic; improvement occurs in all children, learning-disabled or not.

The new approach is to try to define the causes of a learning disability and remove them if possible, and to design a teaching programme tailored to the capabilities of each child. Such an approach requires a multi-disciplinary team comprising psychologists, teachers, physicians, speech therapists, audiometrists and orthoptists.

Conclusion

We hope that a clear message comes across in this chapter and section: dyslexia is a symptom and not a disease. The second message which we hope is obvious is that dyslexia is avoidable, certainly in a large number of cases.

If the connections between some illnesses and dyslexia are recognized by family doctors, teachers and parents, then appropriate action can be taken very early on and the child's capabilities preserved intact. Prevention is better than cure.

Lastly, reading and spelling are facets of language. Dyslexia is a symptom of a large number of language disorders. Approach it from this angle and it becomes easier to understand and to help than if it is regarded as a discrete entity.

Never ask, 'Is my child dyslexic?' but always ask, 'Why is he like this?'

Summary of Part II:
Prevention rather than cure

If you have made your way through the whole of Part II, you will realize that there are some medical conditions which contribute to school failure, especially among children of lower than average intelligence or who are at risk to learning difficulties because of unsatisfactory environments. Some of these medical conditions can be avoided, with consequent reduction of the risk of learning disabilities developing.

Before you are stricken by nail-biting guilt because you failed to take action ten years ago, remember that the relationship between any medical conditions and learning disabilities is not an inevitable one. Some have only recently been identified as important factors in the dyslexic equation and neither you nor your doctor could have done anything preventative. In some, the responsibility for taking avoiding action is not in parents' hands. Here is a list of preventable conditions which may have an effect on school performance, arranged in roughly chronological order.

Relevant Conditions

Time	*Disease*
Before birth	Rubella
	High alcohol intake
	Lead
Birth	Damage
	Biochemical disturbances
Early childhood	Virus infections
	Recurrent middle-ear disease
	Lead
	Food allergies
	Severe head injuries
	Eczema
	Depressive disease

Early school	Anxiety
	Glue ears
	Threadworms
	Asthma
	Unestablished reference eye
	Nasal obstruction
Later school	Epilepsy
	Drugs for epilepsy
	Short sight
	Uncorrected short sight
	Drugs of addiction

If nothing is done to prevent their occurrences, such medical conditions may lead to changes in a child's capabilities and potential.

Different psychological and physical defects produce different patterns of dyslexia, each requiring different teaching techniques.

So before this or that teaching programme is applied to a child who is failing in school, the underlying medical factors must be identified. Otherwise, the parents and teachers are in danger of attempting to treat only the classroom symptoms without understanding which mechanisms are at fault. Such action is unscientific, to say the least, and at worst resembles inefficiency.

PART III

Chapter Twelve
Reading

A definition

Reading is communication: as the reader thinks under the stimulus of print he re-creates the writer's message. The meaning attributed to the message depends on both writer and reader. In the same way that a writer, whether Tolstoy, Beatrix Potter, or Aunt Maud in her Christmas letter, brings the whole weight of personal experience to the writing of the message, the reader also reads with his autobiography. Take a crude example: Mungo Park's *Travels in the Interior of Africa* is a fascinating book by any standards. But the reader who has travelled from the Gambia through Senegal and Mali will find the book a lot more rewarding than the armchair reader who has never set foot in West Africa.

138

Reading with children at home

The setting

The first essential, without doubt, is to make reading comfortable, a delightful activity in a cuddly setting. From the start, let the child associate the literal warmth of your affection with reading. It is easy to have the toddler in your lap; bigger children can sit on the sofa or on large cushions on the floor, or can even snuggle under a rug if reading comes after some exertion in the cold, like a swimming session in midwinter. Have a cosy light, perhaps a warm drink, perhaps a supply of sultanas that the child can eat absentmindedly while you read to him. Perhaps he'll stroke the cat, or, on a hot day, vaguely dig in the sand-pit while you read to him about Pooh stuck in Rabbit's front door.

139

There's a lot to be said for the traditional daily bedtime story. Another good opportunity is the family holiday, especially during those slow meals with long waits for food. The *Iliad* read in a Greek taverna, where waiters have been known to be called Achilles, takes on an immediacy it lacks in the Anglo-Saxon north. By the same token, *The Hobbit* is just right when rain maroons you in your caravan in the Highlands.

The start, with pictures

140 You will have noticed how very small children enjoy turning over the fat pages of ragbooks. At about the same time parents are pointing to and naming objects, 'shoes', 'brush', hoping that the toddler will repeat the sound and so learn to associate it with the object. If a picture-book of photographs of the same single objects is to hand, these will also be named as the pages are turned. And the child will, very slowly, begin to realize that three-dimensional objects can be represented by two-dimensional pictures.

Your child will also be hearing nursery rhymes; when, a little later, pictures illustrating them are shown to him, the idea will form that a lot of words go with a – for the child – complicated picture and that the main features of the picture correspond to the most important words. Later still, but well before school age, very short stories will be told and tiny books read. Kindly grandparents and the public library will be hard put to it to keep up with demand. The child will develop preferences, asking for the same story over and over again, and if the reader mistakes one word or fails to turn the page at the right moment the child's correction will be swift and unmistakable. The child will have established a firm link between a given picture and a particular set of words, the message being carried by both print and picture. He will also know about the permanence of text.

Stories in print

141 With time, the child will move on to longer and more elaborate stories. They will extend his imaginative range, giving him – at second hand – a width of experience for which real time is too short. They will increase his vocabulary and give him familiarity with the conventions of storytelling. At its simplest, he will recognize 'once upon a time' and 'they lived happily ever after' or 'they went home to tea' as markers signalling the beginning and end of a wide range of stories. These are considerable gains, but parents could be adding another very practical one: while you read to your child from illustrated books, use your finger as a pointer to follow the print. The movement of the finger along the line from left to right and back again ('the return sweep', as the jargon has it), and from the top left-hand corner of the page to the bottom right, will give your child an understanding of the direction of print. If you read with expression and emphasize particular words ('there was such a splish-splash-splorum'), you will find that your child will begin to associate a set of squiggles on paper with a sound/word, and, just as useful, he will realize that the gaps between the squiggles mark the boundaries between the groups of sounds/words.

Great excitement is generated by stories in which the chief character shares the child's name. Mike, hearing a story about Mike, will identify with his namesake and enter into the world of the story with gusto. This is the ideal opportunity for extended conversation about the story (an essential adjunct to reading): what is likely to happen next? why did he do that? would the real-life Mike do things in the same way or differently from story-Mike? how could the story develop or end, and who are the goodies and the baddies? Real-life Mike may well decide to tell his own version of the story, or invent one from scratch. Try to write it down (if possible, type it), cut pictures out of magazines with Mike's help, make a little cover and give him his own book. He will then be 'the onlie begetter' of a complete story, which may well alter on subsequent 'readings', showing that reading is the re-creation of the author's message. At what age of child should parents stop reading to him? As late as possible, preferably as long as the child is not reading to himself for pleasure but willing to listen while he makes models, mends his bike, plays patience. Even if he does read for fun, there will be books which are a bit too long, or too difficult at a particular stage of his reading progress. If it is a favourite of yours, why not introduce him to it? Fashions in books change: these days, not that many ten- or eleven-year-olds choose to read *Kim* and yet thoroughly enjoy it if it is read to them. With a bit of editing and a suitable tone of voice, *The Castle of Otranto* goes down well – good as a half-way house between a joke and a horror comic, and an excellent starting-point for family discussions about horror films and books.

Think back to the books you enjoyed, browse round the children's library and consult its catalogue (you'll be surprised at what is kept in the stacks). You are sure to find something he will enjoy. But most of all, enjoy it yourself; speaking from personal experience, reading to one's children is one of the major pleasures of parenthood.

Before school

Recognizing reading and writing
One of the ways that a child learns to speak, and so make sense of the world, is by labelling objects. 'Table,' says Mum, pointing to the coffee table. 'Table,' says Dad, pointing to the kitchen table. 'Table,' says

142

Gran, pointing to the dining-room table. It takes a while for the toddler to abstract the essential features of the objects, to realize that the one sound refers to a variety of tables, that objects placed on them do not detract from their essential character and that they can be put to a large number of uses. To understand the term 'table' the child must recognize the object and remember its uses, that is, put the object in its daily context.

Recognizing a process visually as varied as reading is a lot more difficult than recognizing the 'table-ness' of all tables. But your child should be able to recognize it before he starts school. So it needs to be specifically pointed out. You may like to try some of the suggestions below:

1. Before you cross the road at a pedestrian crossing, press the button and if the word WAIT lights up, point it out.

2. When you are trying out a new recipe, read out each step ('Beat four egg yolks with the sugar') just before you do it; do the same with DIY equipment, instructions for model-making, sewing or knitting.

3. Read out the names on cereal packets, tubes of toothpaste, etc., the 'serving suggestions' on tins of food, the ads on TV.

4. Read out the signs in shops ('Frozen foods', 'Cash desk', 'Escalator') and the names on the bags given by the shops.

5. Point out the notices in the street ('Bus stop'), in the park ('Keep off the grass'), street names and house numbers, posters for coming events.

6. Don't forget clocks and dials (in the car, on the boiler, on the cooker).

7. Explain why you are reading parts of a telephone directory, train timetable, menu (and later, maps and dictionaries).

8. Make a point of consulting with the child a paper or magazine showing TV programmes, a book of information about something of interest to him (cars, birds); show him and read to him from the local paper if there is a piece about something he has noticed locally (a house being pulled down, a new filling-station, etc.).

9. Read to him holiday postcards or birthday cards from friends and relatives and tell him about letters you may have received from them.

10. Read to him, for his and your own delight [141].

You are sure to think of a great many other instances, daily.

When it comes to writing, the case is somewhat different. For a start, from the age of about two and a half a child will pick up a pencil and scribble with great enjoyment, though of course he won't know the difference between writing and drawing. By the time he is five he should recognize without trouble the difference between a drawing or photograph on the one hand, and print or handwriting on the other. The act of writing is probably easier to recognize than the process of reading, because there are three visible elements: the writer, the writing tool (still mostly pens and pencils, sometimes typewriters and VDU screens) and the finished product – a sheet of paper covered in what is recognizably not a picture, is most often handwriting or at least some handwriting among the typescript. And writing tools and the finished piece of writing are not, to the non-reader, as varied as the innumerable sources of reading matter.

Again, a child needs to know why writing is done. As you write, it is a good idea to specify: 'I am leaving a message for dad/don't want to forget that address/telling gran what we did yesterday/saying thank-you for my present/making a shopping list/telling a story'. If your child wants to send a message to gran, ask him to repeat it while you write it down: 'Moggie's had three kittens and they keep their eyes shut all the time.' Read it back to him, pointing out each word in turn. You may have to repeat the pointing and explaining, as you write and then read, time and time again before the reasons for writing are well and truly grasped. To sum up, by the time your child is six at the outside he should have no doubts whatsoever about recognizing:

- reading behaviour (what it looks like when someone is reading);
- objects from which reading is done;
- reading material (print of various types and sizes, handwriting, dials, and so on);
- writing behaviour;
- common writing tools;
- the written product.

It goes without saying that he should also be able to enumerate about half a dozen uses for each process.

The conventions of print

With your five-year-old all agog for school or kindergarten, you will watch him buzzing off each morning for the fun and excitement of new friends to play with, fresh materials to handle, novel activities to try. All unknown to himself, he will be starting to read, too. Soon he will

143

realize that the teacher is using words to do with reading and that maybe he doesn't quite understand them. Confusion, misery and sulks can follow only too easily, but fortunately parents can untangle a large part of the trouble. Does your child know the words 'print', 'printing' and 'writing' (in the sense of handwriting), and can he distinguish between the two? Of course he can, as long as you have done what was suggested in the earlier section [142]. Can he tell the difference between a number and a letter? Very likely, if you have followed the suggestion in the same section. Can he point to the top and bottom lines on a page of print? Yes, certainly, if you have been playing and talking with him, teaching him the words 'top' and 'bottom', and have been reading to him. Can he point to the top left-hand corner of the page as the spot where one starts reading a story? Can he run his finger along the line from left to right, with the return to the left for the start of the next line, to show the direction of print? Certainly yes, if you have been reading to him as we suggested. He will also know that the left-hand page is read before the right and that, except for strip cartoons, the print rather than the pictures carries the story.

If you have been reading to him in the way we suggested, he should be able to point to one word, two words, the first or last word. If he has had a shot at writing his name, he will know the difference between a word and a letter, should be able to recognize capitals at least by their size and know that names start with them.

In due course you can help him to distinguish sentences from words (for which he will need to recognize full-stops and question-marks) and relate capital letters to lower-case ones.

Why should parents go to all this trouble? Because children who come to school with a good grasp of the purposes of literacy, what it looks like to be reading and writing, and with a knowledge of the terms used in learning to read and write, make significantly faster progress with reading than those children who lack this basic information.

Summary (138–43)
Parents should start reading to the child when he is very young; they should continue reading to him and talking about books until he is adolescent; they should continue talking about books throughout his schooling.

It is a very good thing if a child starts school recognizing reading and writing, and knowing why they are done.

A child will learn to read faster if he starts school knowing the conventions of print.

Reading in infant school

Starting

If you listen to the conversation of five-year-olds you realize that their language is firmly egocentric. They are not aware of language as such, even less that it might have different functions and techniques, let alone problems. For them, reading is an activity performed almost entirely by adults, divorced from themselves until their individual self-awareness has brought them to realize, each one for himself:

144

1. I do things and I can think about what I'm doing.

2. I can talk about what I'm doing, or have done, and so I can share the doing when I'm face-to-face with others.

3. I can record what I'm doing and through the record share my doing with others even when I'm not on the spot.

4. Other people can record their doings and so share them with me.

This realization marks a considerable development of both self-consciousness and the demands of other people. You, having read to and with your child and written down his messages, have brought him to this realization by his fifth birthday.

In school, the first essential is talking in a friendly way with the aim of sharing experience; real live experience brings fresh material which, once it has been consolidated by talk, is material for recording. Supposing the kitten climbed up the tree, couldn't get down and Dad had to climb up to bring it down. The child chats about this in class, draws a picture of the event, takes it to the teacher and dictates to her: 'Pussy climbed up the tree.' She prints the caption under the picture and the child either traces over or copies the letters underneath and reads the sentence back to the teacher. The child's own experience and language are used to construct his personal reading materials, for these daily pictures and captions are assembled by the teacher into the child's personal 'book'. Gradually the child will try his hand at writing his own captions. At this stage teacher may ask, 'What word would you like to learn today?' The selected word, with intense personal meaning (so it is likely to be a noun or a verb) will be written on a card, taken home, learnt (with luck!) and returned the next day. As a result, each child will be building up his personal reading vocabulary, ideally at the rate of five words per week.

At the same time, the children in the class will have shared a number of experiences in school: they will have drunk milk, listened to stories, counted blocks, cut up paper, painted pictures, looked at books, made things out of plasticine/wood/cardboard, dressed up for 'pretend games'. The teacher will assemble pictures of these activities, preferably by photographing the children engaged in them. The pictures/photos will be given captions: 'We are drinking milk/painting pictures/cutting paper/playing hospitals', and assembled into a folder. This is left accessibly on a table, so that any child can look at it and read the captions. And they do, very gladly, look at the pictures of themselves and their classmates, and read the captions to themselves. The point of this, apart from reading experience, is to demonstrate that shared experience leads to a record equally valid for the whole class. It is also a way of drawing attention to words which are necessary for further writing and reading, but which the children, individually, may not have selected for their personal vocabularies, words like 'are', 'that', 'of', and so on. These various pictures with captions of sentence length do not amount to a story with a beginning, a middle and an end.

Making and reading stories with friends

145 Every day the teacher of a reception class will tell or read a story to her class. (If, on return home, your child wants to re-tell teacher's story at unconscionable length, try to remain interested. The length, with luck, is due to his additions [199].) The teacher will also ask the children to tell a story. This is done individually, or in groups, using puppets or cut-outs, sometimes acted. The story is turned into a book, with pictures from magazines pasted into a scrapbook, telling the continuous story written with teacher's help. The child's own writing at this stage may well be strings of letter-like forms, with occasional gaps: this shows that he has grasped the difference between words and letters, an important step. If he knows some letters he will use them for his own version of spelling; this will tell you that he knows the difference between letters and non-letters, another significant milestone. In these 'books' pictures and story have equal importance [141]. A cover is made, a title chosen and written together with the names of the collaborating authors.

The printed books a child tackles in infant class are sometimes extremely large, with correspondingly enlarged print. These are intended for shared reading: three or four children join in 'reading' the text of a familiar nursery rhyme; they use the gaps between the words to locate any particular word by checking off from the start of the sentence. This is the matching stage of reading, that is, matching a spoken word with a group of letters which are not individually known. Sometimes giant versions of the earliest books of a reading scheme are available in this type of collaborative effort, when the most advanced pupil will be able to find the same word if repeated on a page of print.

Reading in pairs presupposes that two children between them have more sophisticated skills: some words are remembered as long as they are in context, which in turn means that the sequence of words can be predicted from meaning (partly derived from familiarity or pictures accompanying a new text) and syntax; most letters will be identified and named, which leads to finding words that begin with the same letter, and possibly even end with the same letter. In due course this skill extends to unfamiliar pages; gradually letter sounds are learnt. This is useful for self-correction of reading, or, with the help of meaning, prediction of unfamiliar words. By now, all letters as written will be fully identifiable and copying accurate. Given a number of words on little cards he will be able to assemble them into sentences and will know what other words are to be added to make a comprehensible personal message.

Later still, context and grammatical rules, as well as sound–symbol association, are used to identify words; endings like -ed, -ing, -s are recognized and correctly interpreted. Out of context letters are associated with sounds heard at the beginning, end or in the middle of words.

To achieve all this on the way to independent reading in the crowded years of infant schooling, two approaches are used: reading schemes (of which more below) and the 'natural approach'. The latter involves grouping all the books in the classroom (and mostly 'real' books at that) into three or four levels, colour-coded for difficulty, and the child browses through the books of each level in any order he chooses. This approach has great advantages:

- the child's pleasure in reading is enhanced, not least by his control over his progress;
- wide experience of books of genuine quality, with natural language, variety of story line and story-telling conventions from a diversity of cultures; consequently
- avoidance of the contrived language forced on the author by the structure of a reading scheme, and avoidance of the deadening monotony of one author only, in her good and less good moments – and there are inevitably a great many less good ones ('When I hear of another lot of books by X I reach for my gun' has been said by many an infant and junior school teacher.)
- experience of a variety of illustrations, type faces, styles of presentation;

– any and all appropriate books, as and when they become available can be used.

This enriching approach, designed for delight in reading, works well if:

– there are a great many books;
– reading aloud and discussion of the book is done by each child daily (repeat daily), either in school or at home;
– informed parents co-operate actively;
– in school a great deal of writing is done and corrected;
– school implements a well structured spelling programme;
– the child attends school regularly, has no learning disability, an IQ [67] in the average range or above, and speaks English well.

Some infant schools start using reading schemes from just about the first day, with the aim of getting everyone reading in the shortest possible time. Other books are available for private reading or taking home, but their use, while encouraged, is entirely voluntary.

Summary (144–5)
The child starts reading by talking, drawing and writing about his experiences.

Telling and re-telling stories and making up picture books with captions is a friendly way of developing language and reading.

At the start a child learns to read by writing his own stories and reading about his own experiences.

Beginning readers are often most successful when doing so in groups or pairs.

It is possible, and very enjoyable, to learn to read without using a reading scheme.

Reading in junior and secondary schools

Reading schemes

LANGUAGE EXPERIENCE

146 A language experience scheme consists of jolly booklets on topics such as a child might encounter in his daily round. Words appropriate to the situation are used; the child's oral language, knowledge of the situation depicted and interpretation of the pictures should largely see him through, certainly in the early stages. Gradation is achieved by total length, complexity of syntactic structure and use of words known to be in the vocabulary of the average child at a given age. At any level of difficulty, any one of several books of that degree of difficulty can be read in any order. Clearly these are loosely structured schemes, excellent for the child with good oral language and reasoning powers; each book is a 'proper story' with a climax and conclusion, one or two are even poetic, and a high proportion are books for delight. These schemes are underpinned by a device called a 'sentence-maker'; this is a folder holding a number of cards, each with one word – from the reading booklets – printed on it. By manipulating these cards and adding others of his own choice the child can compose, alter or extend sentences or tiny stories before copying them into his exercise book. This ties in with teaching spelling as part of purposeful writing [177, 178]. The sentence-maker, which was put into circulation some years ago, can now be seen to have another use, that of an introduction to word-processing, where some programs contain lists of the commonly used words. It can be used as a spelling aid, and words can be shifted around with ease.

VOCABULARY CONTROL

147

Vocabulary-controlled reading schemes based on look-and-say principles are, as the name suggests, meticulously controlled. A small number of words will be introduced in the first book and repeated – to the adult and to some children *ad nauseam* – with a variety of illustrations, until sheer repetition drives the image of the first sixteen or so words into the visual memory. A second booklet, with the same vocabulary differently deployed and with fresh illustrations, may be available. The next book will repeat the first sixteen words and introduce another six or seven, and so on. These schemes are systematic, repetitive, have no real story-line and they are often deadly dull. To counteract these disadvantages, some reading schemes try to accommodate a story-line which leads to an extension of vocabulary. Since a bigger vocabulary is more difficult to retain, adventitious aids may be brought in: the characters from the stories may first appear in the classroom as figurines. 'Here is Roger Red Hat,' says the teacher, showing the toy to the child and hoping that when, a little later, the child comes to the first reading book he will recognize the figurine on the first page and echo: 'Here is Roger Red Hat.' The system breaks down if the figurines get lost, broken, daubed with a different colour, or the child just takes a dislike to one of them and distorts the opening sentence with demotic additions – risks ever present in the real live classroom.

These particular hazards are avoided in a reading scheme originating in New Zealand: a strictly controlled core vocabulary can be added to in every booklet by so many words made explicit by illustrations and a smaller number of words that will not be illustrated. The second group of additions must be carried forward into books of the next level of difficulty, and so on. This structure lends itself to a considerable variety of 'proper' stories, and so, together with the language experience reading schemes, gives children an early taste of different story-telling styles in print, an important extension of literary experience.

PHONIC SCHEMES

148 Finally there are phonic schemes, based on phonic analysis and synthesis. Reading books in these schemes are also graded by total length, but primarily by sound–symbol association of the letters making up the words. So the earliest readers will have words consisting of consonant – short vowel – consonant, like 'cat' or 'dog', and the next readers will have a few words with consonant blends, like 'desk' or 'ink'. The stories or booklets will gradually work their way through consonant blends ('bl', 'sm', 'cr', 'tw', etc.), digraphs ('sh', 'ch', etc.), go on to vowel blends ('ai', 'oy', 'ea', etc.), and so on. The first trouble with phonic schemes is the order in which the phonic units are introduced. For instance, one popular phonic scheme puts 'ir' towards the end of the sequence. The question therefore arises: how, in the early stages, do you refer to girls? 'Lass'? 'Popsy'? 'A bit of crumpet'? After contrived language, the second trouble is that phonically easy words, regardless of their other features, are introduced as soon as the phonic gradation allows. This led to the inclusion, in a booklet designed for six- to seven-year-olds, of the phrase: 'I had intended . . .', some way from the spontaneous language in that age group. The third trouble is that a well-taught child, or one of good analytical ability, who can differentiate the letters and relate them to their sounds, often does so at the expense of meaning. Print will be mouthed efficiently, but meaning will be lost.

How reading schemes develop reading

149 Notwithstanding all the above ungenerous carping, all three types of reading scheme contribute to the development of reading: the child's own booklets confirm him in the belief that reading is his language permanently held. The language experience schemes reflect it back to him in extended form so the child realizes that books are someone's urgent self-expression, in the same way as his writing is his individual and equally urgent self-expression; that books can be puzzled out to yield meaning, extracting the experience of the writer to be annexed into that of the reader; and that books are for pleasure. These books are read, in the early stages, accurately and slowly.

Controlled-vocabulary schemes, built round a firm story-line, keep meaning predominant but also give the child whole-word recognition. Look-and-say is 'chunking' by meaning [37]. This enables him to read faster by fixing on those words in the sentence that are important for meaning; speed of reading familiarizes him with grammatical cues. He can then readily use the standard strategy for tackling unfamiliar words: read to the end of the sentence and have a guess in context. This and other strategies arise quite spontaneously from the child's desire to find the easiest and most effective ways of extracting meaning from print.

Phonic schemes teach children how to build up words from the sound values of the component letter combinations. The technique does not work if the child has a history of hearing loss [31–7], if his IQ is in the low average range, or if his speed of information-processing is so slow that he loses the meaning of the whole while trying to build up the parts. But if he can quickly – and the emphasis is on quickly – sound out the first letter or letter blend, the sound will be another clue (the first being the local context, the meaning of the sentence) to the identity of the word; the end of the word is often a syntactic (grammatical) clue. In practice, an extensive and comprehensive phonic reading scheme is never read right through. But a limited number of phonically-based texts, as long as they are short, humorous and with illustrations to match (like the 'Dr Seuss' books), will be a useful tool for any teacher of reading. Phonics are primarily useful for spelling, by means of games, crosswords, etc.

All three types of reading scheme contribute to the problem-solving nature of reading because they all, to a greater or lesser extent, apply the child's reasoning ability to understanding the relationship between spoken and written language. Therefore a school with a well-thought-out language policy will have books of all three types in the classroom. But it is important to remember that, in the early stages, the child progresses with reading at least as much through his writing as through his reading. Understanding of this close link is leading to much wider use of the 'natural approach'. With this, only 'real books' are read. The classroom has its own mini-library, where a variety of books will be grouped for difficulty and the groups colour-coded for ease of administration [158]. The natural approach enhances the pleasure of reading by giving the child more choice. It avoids artificially constrained text and gives wider experience of language, styles of story-telling and illustration; these are great aids to reading and talking about reading. Children whose reading progress falters because of limited oral language often gain from this approach. For them it has the additional benefit of camouflage: they are following the same routine as their more proficient peers.

Conventional wisdom sometimes says that if a child is having difficulty learning to read, a highly structured scheme (look-and-say or phonic) should be used to teach him, on the grounds that the child needs to be specifically taught every tiny step. The teacher will know what has been taught, what has been retained and what needs to be taught next. Inevitably this amounts to a slog, with variable results. It takes an unusually good and well-equipped remedial teacher to provide a variety of reading within a tight structure.

Increasingly, computer programs are used to help the halting reader. As long as the child has no visual problems with reading off the vertical monitor rather than the horizontal book, the approach has several advantages:

- the excitement of operating the word processor serves to hold the child's attention and greatly improves his motivation;
- programs are interactive, so the child's response, by keying in answers, commands and choices, becomes the writing component that underpins reading;
- the programs are often adventure stories, involving problem solving and logical thinking based on close attention to text and graphics;
- the scope for painlessly correcting, editing and printing out is a great comfort to the child who is still too slow to obtain pleasure from his competence with reading and writing.

Children with reading difficulties often take much longer to reach take-off speed; they find it hard to retain over the holidays what was learnt during the term. If your child is having extra reading, in or out of school, and then in the summer break he does no reading, writing or word games for six weeks, don't expect to be popular.

One general rule to remember: a child who reads regularly at home, who is read to, talked and played with, will make better and faster reading progress than one who does not have this form of parental support. In this particular corner of language development, as for language overall, the potential for parental contribution is crucial.

Beyond reading schemes

150 Most reading schemes peter out when the texts reach a 'readability level' (R L) [158] of about 10, though a few go on to 12. But after R L 10 the demands of the school curriculum and expanding horizons call for a considerable increase in vocabulary, too varied to be accommodated within a reading scheme. Phonic knowledge may help a youngster to get his tongue round words, and word games can be fun, but talking – sociable, purposeful, informative – with adults and peers is the basis of further progress. Build on it by just reading more.

But if your child is still in junior school and has already read his way through the graded readers of one or more reading schemes, he will next be 'on library'. This will consist of the normal, commercially available children's books, and the quantity to choose from will depend on school policy and the generosity of the Parent–Teacher Association. If there is a family reading group [157], join it, or combine with other parents to start one.

At home, you must ensure that he has plenty of absorbing reading matter. You will have to comb public libraries, 'swop shops', jumble sales and bookstalls to find 'good literature', the blessing which Dean Colet of St Paul's, founder of the school, prayed that all children should be granted. Help your child with these 'stretching' books, which will nourish and parallel his expanding horizons. Extended silent reading of nourishing material will strengthen his feeling of personal identity.

But, you may say, 'He's gone off fiction.' Certainly boys more often than girls read for information only. You may have to show him how to use an index and table of contents, and teach him skimming (akin to rapid forward wind) until he homes in on the key phrase and fans out from it, to pick out the precise gobbet of information he is after.

SQ3R and other techniques

For reading extensive passages of expository prose and trying to absorb the information, there is a useful routine known as SQ3R:

151

> Survey: Look at the pictures, title, main headings; try to remember anything else you have heard, seen or read on the subject; try to predict the sort of information you will find in the passage.
> Question: Turn each heading into one or more questions. If the heading is 'Rainfall', the questions may be: When does it fall? How much falls? Where does it fall? Does it fall as showers or persistent rain? Is there any hail?
> Reading: Read the text, find the answers to these questions and tease out the other items of information included.
> Reciting: Look away from the book and think over the answers.

How do they fit in with previously known information? Or earlier personal experience? This is where individual judgement comes in.

Reviewing: Go back to 'Survey' and reconstruct the whole in your mind.

This is, writ large, the method unconsciously used by the efficient reader: in reading for meaning he tackles the start of the paragraph and straight away formulates a tentative interpretation about the material to be read; as he reads on he confirms, rejects or modifies the interpretation in the light of semantic, syntactic or stylistic constraints. S Q3R is a technique that encourages reflective reading, with obvious application to revision for exams and useful whatever text the reader is dealing with.

If S Q3R is applied to fiction the reader is also expected to suggest interpretations of the ideas implied by the text, again in the light of his knowledge and personal experience. In the classroom this is the opening for discussion. Teachers also use the technique of analytic study of a text. This is always a collaborative exercise which, through text-based discussion, aims to:

1. identify the key elements of information contained in each section of the passage to be studied;

2. tabulate them so that the reader has a graphic (often diagrammatic) representation of the gist of the passage (very useful for memorizing);

3. extrapolate from the information obtained to ask other relevant questions and consider wider but still related topics suggested by the passage.

As a means of getting youngsters to read reflectively it is efficient and enjoyable.

Computer-based programs designed to re-create a short text, often a poem, are also enjoyed, mostly perhaps by youngsters labelled 'remedial'. Certainly the format includes a competitive element, with the readers – because it is again a collaborative exercise involving constant discussion – trying to beat the computer (itself a powerful extender of concentration span). The programs call for explicit search for meaning throughout (processing of print is eliminated) and it takes the readers, or rather the re-creators of the text, neatly through the semantic, syntactic and stylistic layers making up the whole.

Summary (145–50)

   A child's reading will develop with his writing and with the type of reading scheme used: language experience, vocabulary control, phonic.

   A school with a well-thought-out language policy will teach reading with books of all three types.

   The wider the choice of reading books available, the better for the child's reading.

   Reflective reading and extended silent reading should be well-established habits before transfer to secondary school.

   Reading cannot be separated from listening, talking and writing. The four add up to the way we communicate with each other and with ourselves.

Reading in cooperation with school

Schools

'Parental involvement is the key to reading progress, even in areas of acute urban deprivation' (*Guardian*, 9 October 1984).

152

   In Great Britain, some education authorities leave it to the individual schools to decide whether to involve parents in their children's reading, and if so, how. Other local education authorities suggest policies that should be followed by all junior schools within their jurisdiction. So it may be that one day, when you are collecting your six- or seven-year-old from school, his teacher starts chatting about his progress and asks whether you'd like to, and have time to, help him with his reading. If the initial approach is individual and informal, a direct link between class teacher and parent, continued contact is expected to be individual and informal too. You and the teacher will have to find time to chat every now and again, just to keep an eye on progress. Home collaboration may consist of your child regularly bringing home his current reading book, to read a second time at home what he has read that day in school and perhaps reading a little bit ahead. A record should be kept, by both parent and teacher, of what has been read at home. This type of very informal cooperation has been found especially effective with children who are failing to get started with reading.

   Many schools prefer a more structured approach. Parents are invited to an 'open evening' explicitly designed to tell them about the school's reading policy and inviting them to collaborate. The advantages of this approach are that more fathers join in; that various approaches to reading can be described and discussed; that parental opinion can be canvassed on how they and teachers are to keep in touch; and that teachers get a better idea of how parental interest can be maintained, even in the holidays. For until children reach a certain level of competence they forget in the holidays what they learnt during the term.

Parents

153 In England, helping with your child's reading is seen as a high-status activity and parents express satisfaction at being involved. The task gives parents and children a focus for a structured relationship. Both sides know what is expected of them, both sides know that the task is of limited length (about ten minutes daily). So both can settle down to it: the child to enjoy his parent's undivided attention, the parent to enjoy building up his child's competence. Other things being equal, a child learns very rapidly from a parent, probably because prolonged contact has led the child to understand and respond to his parents' signals. From them he can very readily pick up directions and suggestions, while he may not be able to do the same from his successive class teachers. Also, since one of the ways of learning to read is by reading, just sheer extra practice contributes to increasing ability. Success provides further encouragement. Research has confirmed casual observation: children who read with their parents not only progress faster but maintain their lead even after a formal home-reading programme has come to an end.

In case of trouble

154 Reading can, like food, become a battleground between parents and children. Your child may be unable to accept what both parents are offering and so prefer to read to mother only, perhaps because he wants to maintain his status as a baby; or he may wish to read only to a 'special reading lady', or to his teacher. Teacher and lady are both at one remove from what are perhaps pressing difficulties at home. Teacher focuses on him, provides a safe and private place where, by choosing to read stories matching his own problems (a death, a danger, etc.), he can safely explore them and build up his self-confidence. By getting involved in the story he gains self-knowledge, and as a result he should be better able to live with his parents and face the world.

If your child absolutely refuses to read to and with you at home, don't despair. Tell his teacher and ask her to recommend some games instead. There are many on sale, and indeed some teachers make their own. You may be able to borrow some, perhaps from a specialist remedial teacher. Consult the catalogues of the educational publishers and, perhaps with help from the Parent–Teacher Association, buy a few games, which could be used by other children too. At least one well-known toy shop in central London has an educational games adviser.

Make use of newspapers, magazines and comics. Could he record stories on tape with extra sound-effects? Does he have a toy theatre for which he could devise plays? He may be willing to read to a younger sibling. Try to keep to the daily pleasure spot, reading something to him for his and your own pleasure.

How to set about it

Assuming that both parents and child are happy to read together, hearing your child read should not be an isolated activity. Parents should read to children every day. For verbal dexterity there should be nursery rhymes, jingles, puns, riddles, jokes and phrases from advertisements. Out in the street, instances of print should be observed. Using the *TV Times, Radio Times* or the newspaper for selective viewing should be a joint activity and, after having watched it, the programme should be discussed. The parent should see that there is a stock of books kept for information and pleasure. At the public library there should be plenty of time for choosing the book (choice is the indispensable ingredient of reading for pleasure, the state you are trying to promote), discussing the pictures, the cover, and the print if it is strange. Hearing your child read will fit comfortably into a general aura of literacy.

155

You must next find out how his school and class teacher want you to set about the actual reading. A precise technique may be advised, for instance paired reading. With this, adult and child read aloud together from a book chosen by the child, who signals when he wishes to read alone. Mistakes are noted but not discussed: the correct word is supplied. The method focuses on success. Or the school may want parents to organize a 'book swop shop', useful at any time, most of all when funds are short.

Two very different series of books, designed for parents and children at home, very gradually introduces children to paired reading, to be started with children aged about four. Instructions are given in each book. *Read Along* is funny and mildly phonic. The other, from Ladybird, comes in five tiers with tapes and much decorative paper. Its danger may lie in hurrying through the five stages of difficulty in order to 'bring him on with his reading'. So before you lash out, talk to his class and head teacher. They may prefer you to read books by a variety of authors, to give your child experience of different types of story, styles of story-telling and language.

Guidance

156 More likely you will be given by the school, as well as the books to be read, general guidance under half a dozen heads:

1. Keep the reading session short, no more than ten minutes.
2. Give lots of praise – lay it on with a trowel.
3. Be ready with lots of talk: discuss the situation and the characters, predict the next event, help him talk himself into a fuller understanding of the story, discuss the relation of the pictures to the story and the appearance of the book.
4. Make it enjoyable, not least because you are rewarding his verbal effort with your sustained attention.
5. For words that are stumbled over:
   (a) you could say nothing for a count of five or even ten (to give him a chance to puzzle it out) and then provide the word;
   (b) if he asks, you could provide the word with no more ado;
   (c) you could help him guess the unknown word from the total meaning of the sentence or story (he will have to read to the end of the sentence) with the sound of the first letter as an additional clue; if that doesn't work, give him the word and carry on reading. The aim is for him to get the total message, so the flow of the story must be maintained.
6. Keep in regular touch with the teachers; they will tell you how this should be done. Very often it is by means of a bulletin sheet, with space divided into two for each day: for reading done at home and reading done in school. On this you will note at least the pages at which he started and finished. If the child comes home with a book in which there is more than one unknown word per sentence, make a note of it. The book is, temporarily, too hard for him [**161**].

Family reading groups

157 Many schools run family reading groups, informal meetings at about monthly intervals between parents, children, teachers and librarians. Child and parent come to the meeting having both read the same book; first the child and then the parent talks about it (often a review written by both is also provided). If the book has been read by others in the group they add their opinions. A discussion of other books by the same author may follow. Several books and their illustrations are discussed, a story is read aloud (generally by the librarian) and, finally, books are changed. Parents and children find contact with librarians and teachers much more relaxed in an atmosphere of shared pleasure in reading. Parents and teachers become aware of children's interests and worries, because a situation in a book may encourage a child to explore his own analogous problems and doubts; parents, in commenting on the same situation, can make the family's standards of behaviour explicit. Teachers often consider that reading ability is extended by the increased incentive to read. As always, greater experience of books increases a child's experience, at second hand, of his world and the one imagined by the author.

Using the family reading group, at least one school in England has produced excellent reading lists classified by subject (such as animals, sport, etc.) and reading difficulty.

In general, the stimulus provided by family reading groups is fruitful for bridging the gap between mechanical/functional reading (which is very roughly the reading expertise of an eight- to nine-year-old) and reading at a more advanced level and for pleasure.

It is to be hoped, of course, that reading for pleasure will become a habit. The very able reader of twelve or older should, with sustained interest in books, be able to discuss them and their derivatives on stage, screen and in music, with similarly-minded parents. At the very least, books should remain a focus for relationship between parents and children.

Hard books and easy books

The degree of difficulty of a book is measured by its 'readability level' (RL, for short). This is done by one of a variety of formulae, based **158** generally on the length of individual words and the length of sentences. The latter is obviously a matter for discussion. It follows that readability levels are close approximations rather than precise measurements, but they are very serviceable when used to direct a child to a book that will be within his comfortable, or less comfortable, reading range. A book labelled as being of readability level 8–06 should be read with ninety per cent accuracy by the average reader aged eight years and six months. This average reader's reading proficiency has been measured by one, or several, reading tests, which have been standardized on a cross-section of the normal population [165, 166].

Graded reading schemes start with the earliest reading books at RL 6 or thereabouts, and progress to a maximum of about RL 12. It is rare for one reading scheme to run the whole gamut. However, no reading scheme has enough reading material at every level of readability to provide practice for pupils who are seriously, if temporarily, stuck. Consequently schools use several reading schemes concurrently and back them up with as wide a library as funds permit. Library books which are not part of any reading scheme are still assessable for reading level by the usual formulae. These can be applied to any printed text of sufficient length.

In schools, progression from the easiest books to the more difficult ones is clearly charted. In some cases children have to work their way through one reading scheme before they are allowed to choose any book they like. Reading schemes vary with the changing theories of reading, supported by particular writers and publishers. Alternatively, all the books in a classroom can be assessed for readability and colour coded, so that if a child is making heavy weather of a particular readability level he can sidestep to other books of the same order of difficulty. As a result he gains further experience before moving on to the next. The benefit of this arrangement (apart from avoidance of boredom) is that the distinction between the reading scheme material, library books, books of information, fiction, poetry and magazines is blurred. Children see books as usable as and when needed, in much the same way as particular pieces of kitchen equipment are used for particular tasks.

Levels of reading competence

Independent level

159 A child can read books at this level with ninety per cent accuracy, and derive pleasure and information from them. If the teacher sends your child home with such an easy book, she is probably encouraging him to derive enjoyment from books. She may also be trying to improve the speed and fluency of his reading, to get him to 'put expression' into his reading and to consolidate what he already knows. In these cases parents can, apart from listening to him reading, ask questions about the story, help the child talk himself into a better understanding of it and relate it to his own experience. Even when a child becomes a competent reader he will, every now and again, revert to a book at a much easier reading level. We all do it: not many of us lie on a beach reading Royal Society papers, but a lot of us read thrillers and a few, so help us, romances.

Instruction level

160 Texts at this level are the ones with which a child needs help, at least at first, from teacher or parent. Often the reading book the child is using at school is sent home to be re-read. This is straight revision, combined with an opportunity for the child to say, 'Look what I can read!' It tends to become boring, particularly if something has slipped in class, the teacher hasn't had time to check the child's reading and so he is stuck with one book for the whole term. Parents can help by borrowing books of comparable difficulty and reading these at home. Even a slightly more difficult book is in order, as long as it is chosen by the child and is on a subject of interest to him; if he also has experience of the situations described in it, or knowledge of the special terms used (for instance, the words for parts of a sailing boat), reading will be greatly eased because it will be possible to tackle the unknown word by guessing in the context of his own experience. It is common for children to read books on a hobby which are far in advance (for reading difficulty) of anything tackled, at the teacher's suggestion, in class. At home, you could further encourage your child (particularly if it is an exciting story he wants to get to the end of) by reading alternately with him, sentence by sentence, paragraph by paragraph, or page by page. Or, if it is a long book that you are trying to finish to a deadline, he can read a sentence and you can read a paragraph, or he can read a paragraph and you can finish the page.

Sometimes a child brings home a book at a new reading level, which his teacher has not had time to introduce him to. Start by reading the first few pages to him while he follows the print with his finger and turns the pages. In the usual way, discuss the story and predict possible events, even words. Then let him have a go at reading and tell him the words he does not know. But stop reading every few pages, go back and pick out one of the unknown words. Say to him: 'It says "must" three times on this page. Can you find them all? That's right, it starts with "m". Now you've found another word that starts with "m", that's "map". Can you see "must"? How many letters? Yes, it's longer than "map". Can you see a little word inside "must"? Well done, it's "us".' And so on.

Often a difficult book brought home will be a book of information needed for project work. This is reading for preparation; you may have to show him how to find his way through the book – with the help of pictures with captions, chapter headings, the index – to the part he needs. The danger in these cases is that, having located the paragraph containing roughly the information required, he will copy the paragraph word-for-word regardless of any irrelevant information it may contain, and whether he understands any of it or not. But you can help him to talk about his project explicitly and in detail; you can ask the necessary questions, help him find and consider the answers, and re-tell in his own words as much of the information as he needs, before incorporating it in his written project. This is the start of the habit of evaluative reading, essential for secondary schooling and beyond.

Frustration level

161 Books at this level are totally beyond the child's reading range, even if he is orally familiar with the subject. He may, however, understand and enjoy some of it, if read and discussed with him. For instance, *The Cambridge Photographic Atlas of the Planets*, by Briggs and Taylor, is much enjoyed by children, mostly boys, from ten upwards, but definitely needs selective reading and a gloss from an adult.

Frustration level is avoided if, throughout secondary schooling, reading continues to develop. Longer books are tackled, the language becomes more sophisticated, the literary devices more varied and the ideas more complex. That is, assuming that reading does progress, which is not invariably the case.

A significant proportion of pupils in schools in the United Kingdom get stuck at the level of mechanical reading, represented by texts of readability level up to a maximum of 10, but often lower. For teachers it is easier to get a pupil to that reading level because there are a number of very good reading schemes available, especially tailored to the needs of the teenage reluctant reader. So semi-literacy is achieved, but the gap to real reading power is never bridged. Youngsters who are semi-literate on leaving school generally do very little spontaneous reading. What little they knew in the reading line they forget within about two years of leaving school. Their reading ages, as adults, are equivalent to those of a seven-year-old, or thereabouts. In short, they are illiterate.

Summary (152–61)
Your child's school may run a 'reading at home' scheme. It is a good idea to join it.

Ask your child's teacher about what books your child could usefully read at home, and how best you can 'hear him read'.

Keep in touch with your child's teacher about any reading your child does at home.

Reading regularly at home is a powerful aid to reading progress. The progress is kept up even after a 'reading at home' scheme ends.

Reading tests

Reading readiness

Throughout your child's life he will have his reading ability assessed by formal tests, over and above any informal assessment his teachers may carry out.

162

The first tests will not be tests of reading as such, but tests of reading readiness. These aim to establish how well the child understands the conventions of print [143]. Does he, for instance, recognize 'movement of print' and 'word boundary' (that is, does he know that the gaps between the squiggles on the paper represent the gaps between words)? Does he understand the difference between a letter and a word? Although all these factors can easily be assessed informally, there are two tests in use, Clay's and Downing's. If you are told that your child has been found wanting on either of these tests, ask precisely which items he does not understand. They are easy enough to teach at home, quite unobtrusively.

In a wider sense, reading readiness is governed by neurological development [62, 63, 65]. In school this is manifested, for instance, by his ability to match shapes [65], to control a pencil and scissors [76], to talk with an adequate vocabulary [90] and clear articulation [93], to use a reasonably well-developed syntax [94], and by his readiness to co-operate with the social teaching/learning process [195]. All these can be assessed by separate tests, but the structured observation of the class teacher [105] is just as useful and less disturbing to the child. If in doubt, the infant class teachers can always consult the head teacher and if necessary call in outside advisers.

Criterion-referenced tests

The next batch of tests your child does are likely to be criterion referenced. The earliest ones are often a check on whether he remembers such words as have been taught or have come repeatedly within his field of vision. For instance, in many reception classes some items have labels attached to them: 'door', 'window', 'crayons'. At the end of one term, or two, or three, can he recognize these words when they are separated from their referents, that is to say, the objects they labelled? Does he read 'door', 'window', 'crayons' when he sees the words written on a 'flash card'? Flash cards are held up for a limited time, to see if the child reads them rapidly (in which case he can move on to learning to write and spell them correctly), hesitantly, with self-corrections, or not at all. The teacher will be interested in whether, even at this early stage,

163

he is self-correcting; if so she will be greatly encouraged, because self-correction implies both self-monitoring of his performance and a desire to get it right.

When your child is somewhat more advanced, criterion-referenced tests are useful for checking his knowledge of phonics. How many of the patterns that have been taught does he remember? Has he picked up any others, on the wing, so to speak?

As you can see, criterion-referenced tests have enormous scope. At the time of writing they are becoming more popular. They are one way of checking on the efficacy of teaching, and of keeping a close eye on the progress of individual children in a class.

Standardized reading tests

164 The 'standardized' part of 'standardized reading tests' means that the performance of any child taking the test can be compared with that of the average for his age group.

Standardized reading tests come in two main categories: the oral ones, done individually with the teacher listening intently, and done at the child's pace; the silent ones, often done in a group and often to a time limit.

In a medical context, where poor reading is seen as a symptom, the usable tests are the ones that yield comparable results over a period without being vitiated by practice effect. Reading, and for that matter spelling, tests act as benchmarks to plot the progress of physiological conditions. So the tests have to be usable over several years of elapsed time (as distinct from time as measured by increased reading proficiency).

In general, tests which are more than fifteen years old are considered out of date, because of developments in oral language and theories and practices in the teaching of reading. Consequently the devisers of the tests are constantly updating them.

Some reading tests are set in the context of skills important for written language. This is the case with the reading tests in the Aston Index [104], a battery of tests appropriate for children in primary school. Tests of silent reading comprehension are particularly important for children from the age of nine upwards, because at that age children should be acquiring the habit of extended silent reading for pleasure, information and learning.

A child who takes a standardized (that is, based on an established standard) reading test is given a reading age: a figure of years and months which summarizes his performance. Suppose your child at chronological age 8-10 (eight years, ten months) is tested and found to have a reading age (RA, for short) of 8–10. His reading is up to the national average.

If, after taking the child's IQ [67] into account, his reading is up to two years below his chronological age, he may be said to be backward with reading. If the gap between chronological and reading age is more than two years, he may be described as reading retarded. Notwithstanding these scholarly phrases, there are a few practical points to remember:

1. It is comparatively easy to get a child to a reading age in the 8-06 to 9-06 band. This is substantially mechanical reading. If a youngster leaves school with that level of reading competence, he will be able to read so little that two years later he is likely to have forgotten even more, and so be functionally illiterate.

2. If a school-leaver retains a reading age in the 9-10 band, he can read functionally, that is, for minimum practical needs; he is semi-literate.

3. For the teacher it is a great deal more difficult to raise a child's reading age from round 9 to over 12 than to get him to read functionally. The breadth of reading and conversational demand are, at this later stage, much more important than reading lessons.

ORAL READING TESTS

Oral reading tests primarily investigate reading accuracy, the mechanical ability to mouth print. The test may consist of a list of single words, selected on a basis of frequency of use and word length: so a child at the age of six to seven is asked to read words like 'just', 'girl', 'day', and 'went', while a sixteen- to seventeen-year-old should be able to get his tongue round 'subtlety', 'alienate' and 'poignancy'. These tests of oral reading of single words are nowadays not considered particularly useful, and the less so as the child grows in age and reading competence.

More often the tests consist of sentences, starting with easy ones, sometimes in large print, like 'Come and play ball' (Salford test), going on to 'Delicate individuals should gradually be accustomed to gentle physical exercise' (Holborn test, nowadays old-fashioned) in smaller print. Again, the tester will be noting how the child reads: does he self-correct, and if so, at what stage? As he goes along, or after reading, or at least by looking to the end of the sentence? This would be a sign of the 'psycholinguistic strategy' (seeking to extract maximum

165

meaning from the whole message and then fitting the unknown word into the whole). Or does he try to build up the unknown word by voicing the sound of each letter separately and then putting them together in a continuous sequence? This is the 'phonic approach'. Or does he substitute a word that looks vaguely like the printed unknown word and move blithely on, regardless of the sense?

There are oral reading tests that specifically investigate phonic knowledge: these give lists of words or short sentences which start by containing the simplest patterns of consonant–vowel–consonant ('cup', 'jet', 'run') and through successive stages build up to longer, less common or phonically more difficult words ('puce', 'generous'). There are also ingenious tests designed to assess phonic knowledge pure and simple, where children are expected, on the basis of their knowledge of sound–symbol association, to build up nonsense words like 'mup', 'slet', and so on.

There is an interesting and valuable test of word recognition, the Carver test, relevant for children whose reading accuracy is lower than that of a child of seven years and six months (an age at which a child might still be reading predominantly look-and-say reading schemes). The child has a booklet of five pages, each divided into ten numbered boxes corresponding to ten lines of print, to be successively worked through at a pace set by the tester. The tester gives instructions: 'Look at box number seven. In box number seven find the word "grass", like "the grass is green"; underline the word "grass".' The child has to pick out the correctly spelt word from distractors of gradually increasing resemblance to the stimulus word. If the child does this test in a small group, or alone with the tester, a most valuable insight may be gained into the way the child scans the possibilities and eliminates them one by one before plumping for one particular version.

Since the object of reading is to understand the text, the most useful oral reading tests are concerned with comprehension as well as accuracy. The New Macmillan Reading Analysis (which supersedes the out-of-date Neale) is a very efficient means to that end. It consists of six passages of continuous prose of increasing length and difficulty, and decreasing print size. Each passage is followed by comprehension questions, some literal, some inferential, some calling for a close look at the text or picture, some testing imaginative understanding and extrapolation. There are three parallel forms of the test, repeatable at no less than six monthly intervals and yielding comparable results for accuracy and comprehension. The form on which the test is marked allows for detailed annotation and a summary of the types of mistake made. A detailed analysis of the child's reading behaviour becomes easily achievable. This test is currently being extended to include a batch of mini-texts of the least demanding kind; these will, when fully developed, provide very precise guidance for teacher intervention at the early stages of independent reading.

The Informal Reading Inventory is, as its name suggests, a type of structured observation of reading. It was devised some years ago and has been further developed, mainly by teachers working for the Inner London Education Authority, to become an extremely detailed record of the child's style of reading. Its drawback lies in its very detail: the child's reading has to be recorded and the tape re-played several times for analysis. This calls for much time and great expertise. In the hands of a skilled teacher it is an excellent guide for a remedial reading programme.

The Informal Reading Inventory is also useful for the older, more proficient speller who has trouble with longer words, often of Latin or Greek derivation: syllables are omitted or transposed, reasonable phonic alternatives are used, and some words – once past the first letter – degenerate into scribbles or blanks. Try him reading a passage of similar difficulty. Does he call 'subsequently' 'subsently'? pronounce 'fatigued' as 'fou-tack-yew'? does he balk at 'vociferous'? If so, reading aloud continuous prose of an appropriate level of difficulty may work wonders for both spelling and reading. The unavoidable rallentando in rate of reading provides time for a closer look at the words. This in turn connects the image of the words with their articulation, and the reader hears the sound of his own voice as he follows the print.

SILENT READING TESTS

Silent reading tests are often done to a time limit. The instructions for doing them may be given orally; one practice item may be done with the tester's guidance, so that she can ensure the child, or children, fully grasp what the task involves.

At their simplest, silent reading tests will consist of a series of pictures, each accompanied by several words, and the child has to ring the word that corresponds with the picture. For instance, if the picture is of a tap, the words beside it may be 'trap', 'tap', 'water', and 'slap'. More often, these tests start at the level of sentences: the child has to read a series of incomplete sentences of gradually increasing difficulty in which the missing word – often the final one – has to be selected from four or five possibilities. They start in single syllables: 'Tom put on his door/wall/coat/book/desk', and end with something like: 'The life of a miser is neither sustained by good victuals nor brightened by jovial company; he is the victim of his own generosity/ sympathy/avarice/virtue/curiosity' (NFER test). In some tests the sentence grows into a little paragraph. In others, complete paragraphs (Gap and Gapadol tests) or little stories (London Reading Test) of gradually increasing complexity have deletions of single words, and these words have to be supplied by the child, often with no clues other than those provided by the context of the paragraph itself. In other tests, including some English language O-level exams, longer passages are followed by questions which have to be answered from multiple-choice alternatives, or by writing complete sentences, or by extracting particular words. In these cases, reading and understanding the instructions is part of the test. (The London Reading Test includes one passage of this kind and allows scope for a little free writing too.)

Silent reading tests focus primarily on understanding what is read. They are particularly important for children from nine upwards, when increasingly learning comes through reading, and independent, extended reading at that. In the clinic, the way a child addresses a silent reading test is illuminating. Does he get up, wander about and need persuading to return to the task, or does he return spontaneously? Does he walk out after five minutes, saying either that he can't do it or that he has finished? Does he call his mother to help (or does she go and offer help)? Does he stay put, checking and polishing to the last minute? Is he still writing frantically when time is up, or is he doodling, or staring at the ceiling? So, in the clinic, we are also looking at his ability to get on with a solo task.

In every case, except in public examinations, the tester will be more interested in the way the child achieves his score than in the score itself. Has he filled all the grammatical deletions correctly, but not the semantic ones? Is he therefore a child with correct speech but un-developed language? Has he written in the nearest word that would physically fit into the space? Has he got the tenses of the verbs right? Can he write complete sentences? Can he pick out the required bit of information? Can he rearrange a sequence? His test performance offers clues to the lines future tuition should follow.

His score is converted into an attainment age: if he is CA 9-00 (aged nine) and has an RA 10-06, his reading is like that of the average child of ten years and six months. Sometimes the score is expressed as a quotient or a standardized score. But, to labour the point, the reason for doing a reading test is to find out the child's *style* of reading, and to help accordingly.

Summary (162–6)

For a child of 5+ to 6+ tests of reading readiness, reading and spelling are often replaced by structured observation of what he can or cannot do.

Criterion-referenced tests find out how much of what has been taught a child remembers.

Standardized reading tests of oral or silent reading compare the individual child's reading with that of the average for his age group. They summarize the child's performance with a reading age.

A reading test also pinpoints the way a child reads. For the teacher, this is as important as how much he can read.

The most useful tests of oral reading test comprehension as well as accuracy of reading. Tests of silent reading test comprehension. They are relevant for children aged 9+.

Chapter Thirteen
Spelling

What is spelling?

167 Spelling is the code used to pin down speech; like a fly in amber, meaning is held by the resin of the right letters in the right order. But while we learn to speak without formal lessons, when we come to writing we have to be directed to hear precisely the sounds that make up words. Next, we have to be taught which sounds go with which written squiggle. There's a lot more practising to be done with hand, eye and pen before our written language speaks as directly and distinctly to the eye as our spoken language speaks to the ear.

The ability to do this is not going to be plucked out of thin air. Spelling must be taught and the best way of teaching it is as part of writing for a purpose.

How a child learns to spell

Sound–symbol association

168 When a child starts writing he tells his mother or teacher what he wants to say, she writes it down and he copies it. At first, only two criteria have to be satisfied: (a) that the letters should be recognizable; and (b) that they should be formed with the pencil moving in the direction conventionally prescribed for each letter [190]. The child then re-reads what he has written. If he can point to the successive words as he says them, he is well on the way to grouping written letters into words. This second step is important, because he is identifying the separate words that make up the continuum of speech. He is preparing himself for the next stage, 'whole word' reading and writing, which has to be topped up with phonics before further progress is made. This involves analysis into still smaller units, the association of one sound with one symbol.

Schools have various ways of teaching this. One of the jolliest and most successful is called the Pictogram System, with the letters turned into distinctive characters living in a land of words called

'Letterland'. For instance, 'C', as tradition demands, is a Cat, known as Clever Cat. 'H' is Harry the Hairy Hat Man. If the Cat gets next to the Hat Man, his hat makes Clever Cat sneeze with the characteristic 'ch' sound (never mind about 'ch' as in 'machine' or 'chorus' – we are talking about six-year-olds). Another lively character is W, a Water Witch, whose role is to work out ways of being wicked in words. When she gets next to the Hat Man she knocks his hat off, so the 'H' is silent (bad luck for the Irish). And so, alliteratively, on, offering much opportunity for conversation, story-telling, acting out the brief stories and drawing. This is excellent because (a) it serves to fix the sound–symbol association in the memory; (b) it gets the children talking and listening to phonic instruction with genuine curiosity; and (c) the sounds of the letters are very briefly isolated – mostly they are parts of words, used in various-sized chunks, which allow the child to identify the whole message. This encourages sustained attention to the spoken word.

A productive feature of the Pictogram system lies in its use of the letter sounds as distinct from letter names. This shortens what can be a long and wearisome stage of spelling by letter name. A child at this stage of development often writes Y (pronounced wye) for W (pronounced double you), or G for J. So *just* becomes *gust*, a word often found in the child's spoken vocabulary, and *car* becomes *KR*. If your child seems stuck with this type of spelling cheer yourself with the thought that he has grasped the basic principle that spelling is matching the sound of the word to the sound of some letters of the alphabet.

Continued use of the Pictogram system shows it to be most successful when used from the start, so that even in reception class some conversation can be anchored to the individual letter characters. For older children needing remedial spelling some of the picture combinations may serve as mnemonics, but only as long as the system is not rejected as babyish – a trouble decently camouflaged with one to one tuition. It may, of course, also mask a desire to move on to the word processor.

To return to the beginner: if he makes no headway with the conversational Pictogram approach, it becomes necessary to use tactile and kinaesthetic reinforcement while the sound of the letter is being repeated:

1. The individual letters can be drawn as large as possible in sand or on a board coated in sandpaper for tactile stimulation.

2. The letters can be written very large on a blackboard, or in the air, with whole-arm movement.

3. The letters can be written on the floor and the child walks the shape of the letter in the direction of letter formation (this will involve walking backwards and sideways as well as forwards).

4. The child can lie on the floor in the shape of the letter, with the teacher (or sometimes an occupational therapist, if she is sorting out general spatial confusion) writing the letter round the child.

5. The teacher or occupational therapist writes the letter on the child's back, the child then reproduces it on the blackboard and gives the sound of the letter and a word starting with it.

In short, the teacher or occupational therapist has to find out what the child can do and start teaching at that level [193].

Phonics

169 Phonics is the system that ties symbols (individual letters or strings of them) to their corresponding units of sound, singly or in groups. A large proportion of English words is phonically regular (but you have to know the rules), and, more importantly, a large majority of the words used in the early stages are phonically regular. These therefore become the better embedded in long-term memory, especially if phonics is part of the early curriculum.

If your child's teacher says to you, 'He's not taking kindly to phonics,' ask yourself the following questions:

1. How good is your child's hearing and listening? (See Chapter 3.)

2. How clearly does he speak? Can he speak with pauses between the words? Does he pronounce the ends of words and the constituent sounds of words? [91].

3. How easily can he identify the sounds that make up words? If you say 'mop', can he tell how many sounds there are, or does he have to repeat it with exaggerated spelling pronunciation first? Try saying to him words like 'sun', 'brim', 'rapid' (note that they consist of short vowels and audible consonants only) and see if he can count the number of sounds in them and tell you which the first and last are.

4. How good is he at games like 'I spy'? Does he know any jingles or alliterative phrases? Does he go in for word play? Does he remember nursery rhymes? How about some fresh ones? Remember the popularity of the 'Dr Seuss' books: these are entirely phonically based – rhymes of hilarious absurdity with equally crazy illustrations.

5. Does he recognize rhymes? Can he produce rhymes to common words? Does he specifically realize that rhyming words share a common

element, as in 'hop' and 'mop', although they differ in one element, the first sound?

6. Can he analyse words by sound, so that he can identify words that share the same initial or medial letter?

7. Can he break up longer (two- or three-syllable) words into syllables? (The TV game 'Give us a clue' is a help here.) Can he repeat after you words of three or more syllables?

All the above are ways of using the voice and ear to control the choice of letters to be written.

Using the eye

170

Most children find it easy to analyse words visually, that is, to examine written words for their shared and distinct components, as in 'net' and 'set', 'slip' and 'slap', 'pin' and 'pig'. Therefore, having counted the sounds of a word, briefly isolated them and written a dash for each, the next step is to say, 'What letter do you expect to see at the start of the word/at the end/in the middle?' and write each letter on one of the dashes, rather like playing Hangman. (The teacher will tell you whether she is teaching the letters by sound or by name.) Young children worry 'What is the shape of "e"?' Or 'I know where to start writing "e", but which way round does it go?' Point out that since we write from left to right it is more comfortable if the writing of one letter ends nearest to where the next one starts. Look for the exceptions [190] and make lists of letters that finish backwards and those which finish forwards. More stubborn are the much publicized visual confusion: letters are inverted (turned upside down): 'u' and 'n', 'h' and 'y', 'm' and 'w', 'f' and 't', in descending order of frequency; or they are rotated (turned left to right); the standard confusion is on the one hand between 'p' and 'g' or 'q'; and on the other between 'b' and 'd', and sometimes between all five letters. To young children all these letters look alike, but with time and practice first the 'p' and 'g' or 'q' are distinguished from 'b' and 'd'; then at about the age of eight all are distinguished from one another. Having mastered the distinction, there is a period (even for children who turn into very good spellers) when in moments of stress they revert to the earlier stage and confuse these letters, especially the 'b' and 'd'.

A very powerful aid to distinguishing them is the way in which they are written – the direction of letter formation. Parents are strongly advised to keep an eye on this; although it seems no more than a detail it can, if unchecked, slow down writing and lead to unnecessary spelling mistakes right up to public examinations at the age of sixteen. Therefore 'b' should be written starting with a downward stroke from well above the line; 'd' should be written with the round part first, like 'an "a" growing tall'. Similarly, 'p' should start with the downward stroke stretching below the line, and 'g' and 'q' should start with the round part [190].

Memory for spelling

171 Assuming that the right letters are written in the right order, the correct spelling still has to be memorized. At first each word learnt is unique, but this approach cannot be maintained because it overloads the memory long before an adequate number of words has been memorized. Words have to be analysed for their visual characteristics as they have been analysed for their sounds.

The outline of words can be looked at and the letters thought of in cubist terms. Look at 'lowest'. The outline is like two towers flanking four flat-roofed houses. On the other hand, 'primary' is like two fangs flanking five teeth, and so on. It's fun as a game (the child is given an outline and has to find words that fit), but because one outline can fit several words ('mop', 'cry', 'say', 'wig') it is too imprecise a method for categorizing words into easily memorable groups.

The starting-point for precise analysis is the first letter of the word, then the last. The next step covers the audible consonants somewhere in the middle, explicitly bringing voice and ear to aid the eye. Voice and ear control the next step too, the clearly audible vowels. Finally, there are the silent or near-silent consonants (like the 't' in 'whistle') and the half-swallowed vowels, like the 'e' in 'walked'. Obviously the longer the word the more elaborate the analysis (including division into syllables, looking for little words inside big ones, double letters, roots, prefixes, suffixes, etc.) because more letters have to be processed auditorily and visually before they are aligned in the right order.

Some children persist in having unusual difficulty with spelling [73] with highly prejudicial effects on their schooling. There is one way of cutting the Gordian knot: the child's learning difficulties can be diagnosed in detail and in particular his visual sequential memory can be investigated. If, on the Illinois Test of Psycholinguistic Ability, his visual sequential memory is thirty-six months below his chronological age, or below the ceiling of ten years and six months for children chronologically above that figure, forget about spelling. It will at best, and after gargantuan effort, get to the stage of writing reasonable phonic alternatives, 'wissl' for 'whistle', 'mait' for 'mate', inadequate for public examinations [214].

Stages in spelling development

SINGLE WORDS

'The stayshun is on the opzit syd of the vullee.' This will get you to the station but the writer will not pass a public examination in a language-based subject. It shows that the writer's understanding of spelling has gone through recognized stages, which follow each other consecutively. Poor spellers get stuck at one of the early stages. The child without learning difficulty who is taught to spell will develop broadly as follows:

172

1. The child invents his own letter-like forms, inserts the odd letter or two.

2. He realizes that words consist of letters so his 'words' consist of letters only – any selection in any order without gaps.

3. He realizes that the sounds of words have to be matched by letters, so he writes one relevant letter for each; the name or the sound of the letter may be focused on, and there may be gaps between letters to separate words.

4. He knows that more than one sound has to be represented by letters and he will get the first sound represented correctly; after that he may invent the spelling of the rest.

5. All the initial letters and most of the audible final consonants are identified. If the word is consonant-vowel-consonant he will try the vowel too, but confusion persists, especially between short 'e' and short 'i', as in 'pen' and 'pin'.

6. All the audible consonants, including some consonant blends, are in the right order; in longer words the vowel component of the letter name stands in for the vowel, so 'garden' becomes 'grdn' and 'beetle' 'btl'.

7. He inserts more vowels but only the easily heard ones (so 'house' will omit the final 'e') and the common grammatical markers, for instance the final '-ing' or the plural '-s'. The inventive speller comes into his own with reasonable phonic alternatives ('stayshun' for 'station').

8. He puts in the silent consonant in the middle of words (the 't' in 'whistle') and the half-heard vowels. He knows many spelling rules.

9. He can cope with long words of foreign derivation, he knows the spelling rules or where to look them up, and he knows which words 'look English' and which don't.

In short, English spelling is built on three systems:

– the first – and easiest – consists of symbols (letters) corresponding to sound groupings (phonemes). This is taught through
phonics;

– the second represents grammatical elements; for instance, final
'-ed', variously pronounced, for the past tense;

– the third covers lexical elements, words like 'medicine' and
'medical' or 'consequent' and 'consecutive'.

CONTINUOUS PROSE

173 The length of the written message affects the difficulty of spelling. Is
the child writing single words, one at a time, with pauses in between
and no linguistic connection? This is the level at which, in many schools,
'spellings' are learnt and tested. Phonics will see him quite a way. Is he
writing sentences to dictation? (that is, he is not worried about what he
is writing, the *meaning*, but only how it is to be written, the *code*).
Accuracy even of words learnt by the phonic method drops.

Expand to a dictated passage of continuous prose. Accuracy plum-
mets; the miscues which in sentences might have been reasonable phonic
alternatives or the right letters in the wrong order are now much more
primitive: audible letters and syllables are left out or added, sound-
symbol association starts to break loose.

Try the child on a piece of his own writing, when he has to
decide what he wants to say and in what order, select the appropriate
words, code them into letters, write the letters and punctuate the whole
passage. It becomes an incoherent shambles: words are left out, or run
into one another, or are repeated; their order does not convey a message;
individual words are truncated; letters are doubled or trebled; illegible
scribbles appear in the middle or end and sound–symbol association is
sporadic.

(Note this parallel: children with cerebral palsy can often be
taught to speak in single words. They manage these creditably and
their delighted parents try to get them to speak in longer utterances.
Speech therapists concur. All too often the result is failure and distress
all round.)

Any programme of spelling tuition must include, from the start,
dictations of continuous prose. These will initially be tiny sentences,
incorporating the 'spellings' set for the week, with the surrounding
vocabulary of a similar or lower level of difficulty. Gradually, the
passages will lengthen, the sentences become more complex grammatically, with direct speech included. The set 'spellings' will still
feature and the surrounding text will incorporate earlier ones, as

well as examples of grammatical and therefore also spelling rules. Consequently, the one exercise will give practice with

- the spelling of single words
- the application of spelling rules
- models of grammatically correct sentences
- the conventions of punctuation.

All these are needed for comprehensible free writing, whether narrative, poetic or expository, mastered in that order which also holds good for developing comprehension of various texts to be read.

Spelling tests most commonly consist of dictated lists of words of gradually increasing difficulty. Of these the Schonell test covers the widest range of difficulty. The Peters Diagnostic Dictations are 100-word passages of continuous prose suitable for children from eight to eleven. A dictation is also part of the Vincent and Claydon Diagnostic Spelling Test. In every case, analysis of the miscues is much more valuable than a 'spelling age'. The same applies to miscues in a child's free writing. Spelling tests which are part of particular programmes (for instance, the Blackwell Spelling Workshop) are criterion referenced: they tell the teacher where in the programme to start teaching an individual child and how much he is learning at each stage.

The emphasis of the Vincent and Claydon Diagnostic Spelling Test mentioned above is on the extent to which children have caught spelling on the wing, just by exposure to print. In particular the test focuses on the child's awareness of letter patterns that are probable in English (for instance, the difference between 'tnukuk' and 'miscrible') and his ability to generalize from given letter patterns: for instance, given the picture of a boat and the letter 'b' and the printed words 'coat, stoat, cloak, toast' can the child extract the 'oa' from the four words, remember the audible 't' and combine all the elements to write 'boat'?

Recent use of this test at the clinic reveals at least three distinct groups of poor spellers:

- children who are able to identify the letter patterns needed to build new words (like the 'oa' in 'cloak', 'toast') but cannot add other audible letters (like the 't' needed for 'boat');

- children who recognize when a whole word 'looks English' but are unable to extract the shorter letter patterns (like the 'oa' in 'cloak', 'toast', 'coat') needed for writing new words;

– children who can recognize whether a word 'looks English' (the difference between 'tnukuk' and 'miscrible') but are no good at proof-reading.

The first group benefit from having their hearing investigated – especially their auditory discrimination [103]. Games for the latter may be called for, followed by graded dictation given 'with exaggerated spelling pronunciation'. Articulation should also be checked [92].

The second group need very specific tuition in building up words, starting with searching for visual features that group words into families: hence *rough* and *plough* will be in the same family. Scanning for particular spelling patterns on the page of a book or the column of a newspaper is useful, particularly if the pattern is grammatically determined: 'Look for all regular verbs in the narrative past tense.' Phonic crosswords are enjoyed.

The last group is the most resistant to remediation because their mistakes are likely to be reasonable phonic alternatives [171]. Knowledge of rules helps, for older children Latin is a distinct advantage. Just putting the written piece aside for a few minutes, changing seats or light and then looking at it again often helps younger children.

Further, good cursive handwriting makes no difference to any of these groups of poor spellers. This finding is contrary to earlier clinic experience [192] and generally received teacher wisdom.

The moral seems to be that if your child is a poor speller, don't rush to buy 'the best spelling book' and embark on intensive spelling practice. Have your child examined in detail and a spelling programme devised to suit his strengths and weaknesses.

Types of spelling mistake

174 Spelling mistakes (or miscues) are often another symptom of the particular dyslexia the child may be suffering from:

1. The child with a history of hearing loss may not separate words correctly, or mistake 'm' and 'n', 't' and 'd', etc., or leave out audible consonants, especially in blends (the 'n' of 'bent', for example) or clusters (the 'm' or 'p' of 'empty'). He may get the audible letters, but more often the syllables are in the wrong order, and some may be omitted altogether.

2. The child with poor visual sequential memory may write the right letters in the wrong order, confuse rotatable letters, omit silent letters, double letters incorrectly, write a word correctly on one line

and incorrectly on the next; if he has been taught phonics, he will use reasonable phonic alternatives.

3. The clinically depressed child will confuse rotatable letters, write dashes instead of words, scribble or give up.

4. The anxious child at the start of writing may spell correctly, or at least get the first and last letters of a word right; then only the first letter and in the end he is writing any letter in any order. His performance deteriorates significantly with length.

5. The child with undiagnosed petit mal [120] and the child who has not been taught will make mistakes in any category.

6. The child with poor pencil control may seem to write 'u' for 'a' [191]. Check his visual sequential memory [73] and maths.

7. The child who writes so illegibly that he gets no feed-back from his own writing will be unable to self-correct as he goes along, nor read back what he has copied off the board. Left handers are especially at risk. This will depress performance all round.

8. The child with an unsuspected low IQ may, at the start, get some words right. As writing proceeds his mistakes will become more primitive, doubling of random letters, and scribbles.

Summary (167–74)
Spelling is the letter code used to pin down speech.

Spelling has to be taught and is best taught in the context of writing for a purpose.

English spelling is based on sound-symbol association, grammatical rules and lexical features.

A child's spelling develops through recognized stages from zero to full competence.

Spelling miscues are often additional clues to the learning disability causing them.

Spelling in school

On the wing
Children are constantly in touch with the written word through notices, posters, labels, TV, reading, learning by reading, and various language activities. In all these, children have the opportunity of noting, analysing and comparing the number, shape, size and order of letters in particular words – in short, catching spelling on the wing. In the earliest stages of reading and writing this diffuse approach works – up to a point, and as long as the child has good visual sequential memory [73, 102], good

175

oracy and careful handwriting. It works again in the final stage, when the good speller, recognizing the root of a word and knowing the rules governing suffixes and prefixes, makes an informed, and as it often turns out, correct guess about spelling a word. He will know how to spell 'permissiveness' from knowing 'permit'.

Incidental learning of spelling is not stressful or coercive; it is slow and haphazard. So systematic teaching should be used to supplement it.

Spelling lists

PHONIC

176 To teach spelling systematically, spelling lists are used, with weekly 'spellings' that have to be learnt at home or in school. Lists are based, broadly, on phonic or frequency of word usage principles.

One of the most popular phonic lists was published in its first edition almost thirty years ago. The children are set anything between twelve and twenty words falling into three phonic patterns (for instance, words ending with '-age', words starting with 're-', words ending with 'ice') to memorize in the course of one week, and are then tested. Seven-year-olds start with three-letter consonant–vowel–consonant words; twelve-year-olds have words like 'acquaintance', 'indulge', 'mischievous'. All the phonic patterns are covered over five years and 3,172 words. If the practice of setting, learning and testing is conscientiously adhered to, theoretically the child should, on the eve of his thirteenth birthday, be able to spell the lot. Bully for him!

Much more valuable, especially in schools where a significant proportion of pupils use English as a second language, are methods which combine phonics with word meaning. Again, pupils may be set to memorize a certain number of words sharing one or two phonic patterns and practise using the words in sentences. For testing, the definition of the word is given and the pupil has to supply either the single word or a sentence illustrating its meaning.

With phonic lists, teachers know which group of pupils has reached which group of words, so record-keeping is easy and the next target obvious; phonics can be combined with handwriting, so the child learns to write letter strings like 'ain' or 'ful' rapidly and legibly; the practice of setting, learning and testing provides a routine for classroom management – it is traditional and it doesn't take up too much teacher time. For the pupil, it is certainly easier to learn words that share a sound and a letter string forming a visual pattern than random words, or thematically linked ones like 'pen', 'quill', 'pencil', 'crayon', 'chalk', 'felt-tip' and 'typewriter'. The predictability of weekly setting and testing is often soothing for pupils, and if a class record of spelling progress is kept the child can see how he is coping compared with his peers.

However, the phonic approach has a number of disadvantages. For a start it just does not work for children who are, or have been, hearing-impaired (remember that twenty-nine per cent of children attending remedial classes in London have a history of hearing loss). Secondly, children with limited oral language do not remember beyond the day of the spelling test how to spell words they do not actively use. On the other hand, the child with a particular interest may wish to use an extensive, specialized vocabulary, which will not be included in a phonic programme. And just learning words for 'spellings' week after week becomes downright boring . . .

The teacher recognizes additional practical shortcomings: phonic knowledge is built up progressively, so if a child misses the early stages where the words have a hundred per cent sound–symbol association, he is going to have great difficulty with the more advanced spelling patterns and longer words. And how is he ever going to catch up? Then, few phonic programmes offer the opportunity for practising spellings other than as isolated words and even fewer provide scope for revision and consolidation.

The wider argument in favour of phonics for both reading and spelling is that it provides a general strategy for 'word attack'. The example quoted in a recent publication is that of a child who says the sounds and then reads 'tip', 'top' and 'tap' will also read 'pit', 'apt', 'opt', etc. For a child with a learning difficulty there is a big gap between the two. Having said the sounds of 'tip', 'top' and 'tap', and having learnt to read them at speed and to spell them, he will have to say the sounds of 'pit', 'apt' and 'opt' and put them together repeatedly before he can read the words. He is extremely unlikely to remember 'apt' and 'opt' unless they are part of his spoken, or at least commonly heard, vocabulary; he has a second chance to remember them when they are re-taught as part of the 'pt' group of words (like 'slept' and 'kept').

WORD USAGE – THE RATIONALE

The alternative spelling lists, based on frequency of word use, start from the premise that spelling, or being able to trot out 'spellings' correctly, is not an end in itself. Spelling is seen as part of written expressive language, which in turn is the distillation of the child's

177

knowledge of the world, his attitudes and feelings. Since language is the product of thought, spelling is one way of conveying his thoughts intelligibly.

The words used to convey thought are much the same in all English-speaking countries; the same core of words is used over and over again; for instance, the hundred most common words in print make up something like thirty per cent of all words used by children. But even the most frequently used words are not necessarily easy to spell and therefore cannot be reliably memorized in a particular week of a phonic spelling programme. Further, when the less common of the commonest words in print (that is, not the first hundred, but the second or third) are examined, the frequency of their use will vary with the individual child. So the aim is to provide him with a list of words he personally is most likely to use in writing, to help him focus on such words as he positively needs to learn at any given time, to build in a means of identifying the words in most urgent need of re-learning and to show him how to check his guesses at spelling throughout his schooling.

CLASS PRACTICE

178 In practice each child is set a 'target'. He is directed to words of a particular degree of frequency; for beginners aged six to seven, target 1 comprises 300 of the commonest words, including slight variations of a root word, such as 'doll' and 'dolls'. When in his normal writing a child wants to use a word he does not know how to spell, he has a guess and checks his guess against the word list. This is a mini-dictionary of 300 words arranged in alphabetical order. If his guess is correct, all well and good. If not, he copies the correct spelling from the dictionary into his personal learning list. If the word is beyond his target it is put in brackets to show that it does not need learning yet. Come the end of the week, or the time set aside for spelling, he learns the words from his personal list. Once he knows ninety per cent of the words in his first target, he moves on to the next. As he progresses through the targets his mini-dictionary becomes more elaborate, ending with 2,500 words, each with a number from 1 to 7 beside it indicating frequency of use. If a child working on target 4 finds that he does not know how to spell a word from an earlier target (he may never have used it), he enters it in his personal learning list and underlines it as a reminder that, when it comes to learning, the underlined word is to have priority. Having finished his writing, the child is directed to use his mini-dictionary or personal spelling list for proof-reading.

The benefit of this method is that the child learns the words he

SPELLING

wants to use and is therefore largely in control of his spelling advance; the words are parts of larger units of meaning that he himself has produced. As a result, spelling is seen by him as an integral rather than a discrete skill. The choice of words learnt, those most useful to him, is very likely to keep in step with his developing desire to express himself. Opportunity for revision is built in; so is practice in using a dictionary. Checking guesses is powerfully encouraged (after all, not every word is looked up first, even by the most pedantic child), proof-reading to a lesser extent. Grammatical spelling rules are displayed from the first: the plural 's', the 's' for the third person singular, the '-ed' for the narrative past. Overall the method makes for independence in the speller. Children brought up on this method are much less likely to go to pieces when faced with writing continuous prose.

For the teacher, the drawbacks of the approach are considerable. It takes a lot of time to keep track of each child working at his own pace. His personal learning list has to be checked regularly and testing has to be in small groups. The method is excellent for common words but less good for a personal, specialized vocabulary. It is not appropriate for children with poor visual sequential memories, nor does it lend itself to combining with handwriting (though it is much better to use with a word processor). It depends to a large extent on the child's urge to express himself, on the width of his oral vocabulary, on his goodwill and conscientiousness and, finally, on the care he brings to handwriting. The hand–eye coordination of handwriting will serve to analyse and memorize the disparate words, held in the envelope of meaning of the passage written by the child.

The benefit of this approach to spelling is that it allows the child, perhaps reminded by his teacher, to check his spelling at every stage of written composition. This book deliberately no more than nods at written composition/free/creative writing. But the process may go through the following stages:

1. taking notes from events as discussed or reading, to guide choice of subject;
2. planning the composition;
3. building up detail (including particular phrases) in sentences and paragraphs;
4. writing the final version;
5. revising, proof-reading and perhaps making a fair copy.

If a word processor is used, the following sequence may be followed:

1. as (1) above;
2. writing a first draft;
3. reading the first draft and deciding where changes (including additions and omissions) should come, and how they may be made;
4. writing the second draft;
5. as (5) above, but the printer may take care of the fair copy so that only the format will have to be considered.

School spelling policy

179 It is worth finding out the policy of the school in regard to spelling mistakes (or miscues) in free writing. In a story, a book review or a description, are all miscues underlined or ringed, or is *sp* written in the margin? Or just a few? If so, how many, and on what basis are they selected?

How are pupils expected to cope with words that have been marked as being misspelt? Are the words to be copied out correctly three times, or six times (no good if the child has a poor visual sequential memory)? If it is a grammatical mistake, does the rule explaining the mistake have to be written out, or the whole sentence? Does the entire piece of free writing have to be copied out correctly if it contains X misspellings, or X plus 10, or 20 – or does it not have to be copied out at all? Is there access to a word processor for producing fair copies? Who checks the corrections? What steps are taken to help the persistent poor speller?

Some schools (mainly secondary ones) have explicit spelling priorities, in the sense that all staff who teach language-based subjects agree on: (a) how many misspellings in a piece of writing are to be picked out (this figure will vary with the age and ability of the pupil) so that the whole piece does not end up covered in red ink; and (b) what type of misspelling will justify attention first, second, etc.? These guidelines for marking are then applied by all staff, and pupils are gradually weaned away from the most heinous misspellings, which are corrected first, towards the less important ones.

Imagine a school spelling policy that limits teachers to picking out a maximum of ten misspellings in any piece of free writing, and attaches maximum gravity to misspellings which mask or distort meaning and least to those which preserve meaning. In these circumstances, teachers will look for mistakes of the following kinds, in the order given below:

1. words omitted or inserted that do not fit the meaning of the sentence, or 'words' that are unrecognizable, for example, 'admerle' for 'immediately';

2. words that have had parts of them omitted or added, so that although they are no longer real words their general meaning is clear, as in 'destinitation' for 'destination'. They will also look for mistakes with common homonyms, such as 'were', 'where', 'wear', 'we're';

3. words where endings important to the meaning have been omitted or misspelt. This covers many of the grammatical spelling rules – for parts of verbs and verb tenses, plurals, the formation of adjectives from nouns, adverbs from adjectives, and the comparative and superlative;

4. the right letters of the word in the wrong order, so that (a) they make a word of more or fewer syllables than the original (for example, 'arguing' may become 'aurging'); or (b) the number of syllables stays the same, as in 'field' turning into 'fleid', a very common error;

5. reasonable phonic alternatives, for instance, 'stayshun' for 'station'.

Assuming a child makes fifteen spelling mistakes: none from group 1, two from group 2, eight from group 3, one from group 4 and four from group 5, he will have to correct, in whatever way the school decides, only the ones from groups 2 and 3 and his teacher will notice that his grammar needs further investigation. If a child has seven misspellings all from group 5, he will have to correct them all, and his teacher will wonder whether he was in a tearing hurry, never learnt phonics, or did learn phonics but has a particularly bad visual sequential memory.

Summary (175–9)

To a limited extent, spelling can be learnt through general reading and writing activities.

Most junior schools teach spelling systematically with the help of spelling lists.

Phonic spelling lists tie in well with handwriting practice.

Spelling lists based on frequency of word use teach spelling as part of written expression. They encourage independence in the speller.

A school's spelling policy can, if consistently applied, greatly help a child towards correct written expression.

Spelling at home

SLACAWAC

Your nine-year-old comes home with sixteen 'spellings' to learn. How is he to set about it, with your help? The accepted strategy is S L A C A -

180

W A C, or Say-Look-And-Cover-And-Write-And-Check. (Teachers have been heard to say to their pupils, 'You can slacawac that word.') Bearing in mind that his sixteen 'spellings' could be from either a phonic or a word usage list, look at one of the two worked examples below.

Note: If you are going to help your child with his 'spellings' remember this school habit: letters printed in capitals are referred to by their names, so, for example, H A C is heard as aitch-ay-see; lower-case letters are referred to by their sound, so 'k' is referred to with the same sound as the 'ch' in 'choir', and 'br' does not refer to British Rail.

WORKED EXAMPLE I: PHONIC LIST

181 The chances are that your child comes home with sixteen words written down in a column, as below:

> price
> twice
> since
> fence
> pepper
> copper
> cuff
> stuff
> visit
> fir
> birth
> birthday
> bitter
> silly
> stiff
> hurry

Examine the words for possible ways of categorizing them: two start with 'p', two with 'si', two with 'st', two with 'c', three with 'b', two with 'f'. No harm in writing them down in groups:

price	since	stiff	cuff	bitter	fir
pepper	silly	stuff	copper	birth	fence
				birthday	

Three odd ones remain: 'twice', 'hurry' and 'visit'. Try re-grouping the words, using the longest available letter string as the bases:

price twice	both end in '-ice'
since fence	both end in '-nce'
pepper copper bitter	all have a double consonant followed by '-er'
cuff stuff stiff	all end in double 'f'
fir birth birthday	all have 'ir'

'Visit is the odd man out on both lists. Look at it again. How many letters in the word? Do any repeat themselves? Can you hear them all? Any short words inside the long one?

Now look at this third version of the list again and say the words with exaggerated spelling pronunciation. Pick out any that rhyme:

price and twice   cuff and stuff

Look at 'price' and 'twice'. Are they the same length, or different lengths? How many letters in each? Can you hear five separate sounds? No. Which letter is silent? 'E'. Does 'E' do anything to the sound of the word? It makes I say its name and makes 'C' say 's'. Any short words inside the longer ones? 'Ice'. Without looking at the list, can you spell 'ice'? 'I-C-E'. Say 'price' very carefully (with exaggerated spelling pronunciation). What letters do you expect before 'ice' in 'price'? 'pr'. So the whole word is 'price'. Can you tell me something using the word 'price'? The price of the bus ticket has gone up. Good.

Give the child a wide sheet of paper and ask him to copy the word 'price' 'in best' into the left-hand margin, say the word again carefully, look at it, fold the sheet over so that his writing is hidden. Next he writes 'price' from memory and looks back to check with the original copied version of 'price'. If all is well, move on to the next word. If not, repeat the Say-Look-And-Cover-And-Write-And-Check. Having gone through all sixteen words, as a summary you could repeat the spelling rules exemplified by this list:

1. 'C' followed by 'E' always says 's' – 'price', twice', 'since', 'fence'.

2. In words with a single vowel plus a consonant plus 'e', the 'e' makes the preceding vowel say its name – 'price', 'twice'.

3. But in words with a single vowel plus double consonant plus 'E' the double consonant keeps the short vowel short – 'pepper', 'copper', 'bitter'.

Somewhere along the line the child could also copy out the sixteen words, grouped as in the third list, 'in best', with the significant letter strings in cursive.

WORKED EXAMPLE 2: WORD FREQUENCY LIST

182

clothing
hind
balance
golden
brave
circus
dive
voice
yell
sphere
practice
programme
roar
slipped
expect
lion

Your nine-year-old has been writing about a visit to the circus and comes home with the list above. Again, try to find links for grouping the words:

brave dive	end in '-ve', which illustrates the rule that no English word ends in 'V', and if 'v' is the last sound heard it has an 'E' after it
voice practice balance	both end in 'ICE', and, together with 'balance', illustrate the rule of the soft 'C' (as in the list above)
lion hind	both have a long 'I'. Remind the child of 'kind' and 'mind'. Invent a mnemonic: *Mind the lion's hind legs.*

golden
expect
yell
clothing

are all straightforward, with exaggerated spelling pronunciation. Remind the child that '-ing' is about the commonest word-ending in English, and '-en' some little way behind. Think of words with the same ending.

Exaggerated spelling pronunciation can also be used with 'programme', which can be further discussed in connection with a 'program' for the micro and a 'prog' on TV.

'Slipped' exemplifies the rule of doubling the consonant to keep a short vowel short; compare 'slip' with 'slipper' and 'slipper' and 'slippery', 'dip' with the Big Dipper, 'rip' and Jack the Ripper. Mention '-ed' as a sign of the narrative past tense.

'Roar' begins and ends with an 'R' and is an imitation of the sound a lion makes. An experimental roar is indicated, the word 'onomatopoeia' is not.

This leaves 'sphere'. You could try saying sp-here to show that there is a small word, 'here', inside the longer one; you could mention the sphinx, or the derivation of the word; you could draw a circle and get him to fill it up with the letters of the word stretched to fit, and he could do the same thing round a tennis ball or a football.

And again the words are to be SLACAWAC-ed and a fair copy written out.

Note that older children are sometimes given lists of words for particular subjects to learn. The SLACAWAC principle still applies, but obviously the meaning of the word is crucial.

While the principles used to memorize the words in the two lists above are much the same, the conversation related to the second one is much wider-ranging. Parents may say that the lists should have been examined, discussed, commented on and copied in school. So they should. But your child may not have been in the room when it was being done, or not listening. And will he remember from going through the routine just once? If you are worried about your child's spelling (why else would you be reading this?) then you, or someone on your behalf, will have to go through this routine, or something like it, once a week. Remember this is still the early stage – the spelling of single words only.

More aids to spelling

Word games (Scrabble, crosswords, phonic rummy, etc.) are all fun and they help with single words.

183

For children who find handwriting troublesome, a typewriter at least gets over the difficulty of guiding the pencil in various directions, since only one type of movement, tapping (or gliding with electronic typewriters), is required.

If a long piece of writing is set for homework, there is a lot to be said for first speaking it on to tape and then re-dictating it, playing the tape several times if necessary. This breaks the task in two: the meaning is separated from the coding, so effort can be concentrated first on one and then on the other. A computer with a word-processing program is the greatest help because successive drafts can be made, gradually polishing the product until, in the absence of a printer, an acceptable final version can be copied direct from the VDU. A home microcomputer can be used for SLACAWAC and the weekly spelling lists fed into it, but it assumes some knowledge of programming in the family.

Conscientious children left to their own devices when learning 'spellings' learn, or know, the first letter or two of each word and very often the last one or two also, but have a horrid chasm in the middle. There is no point in devoting effort to already known parts of words; it is better to concentrate on the unknown middle. With a word like 'manufacture' the child can hear and remember 'man' from the start and he probably notices 'RE' from the end, so he needs to focus on 'UFACTU', which has a symmetrical air about it – 'U', then the word 'FACT' with all letters audible, then 'U' again.

There is little point in copying words as a means of memorizing their spelling. SLACAWAC is much more fruitful. But if handwriting also needs to be practised, then words with identical letter strings can be copied, in columns, so that the letter strings are always underneath one another. Add the meaning of the word, or a phrase, to each, as follows:

ever	for ever and a day
every	every boy in the school
never	never say die
very	a very hot day
everyone	everyone listened to the band
everywhere	I looked for you everywhere

This is an extremely good way of practising cursive handwriting, which is one of the main props of sound spelling. There is at least one commercially available handwriting system based on this principle of letter strings; it is very good for junior school children in combining handwriting and spelling practice.

At the time of writing, a very cheerful program called WILT for the BBC-B computer has come on to the market. It is a game (for one or two players) to practise spelling the 400 words most commonly misspelt by nine-year-olds (for instance, 'circus'). Its usefulness lies in encouraging the child to think consciously (and with the help of bar graphs) of the probabilities or frequency with which given letters are sequenced to form characteristic English letter strings. It is a highly interactive program – it does not leave the player just looking at a letter string and relying on visual memory alone.

A recurring difficulty voiced by mothers runs something like this: 'He always has free writing homework (or story finishing) on days when I'm stuck ironing, or sewing, or making bread, and just to get it done in reasonable time I've been helping him with spellings. And now he doesn't seem able to write anything on his own.'

This complaint makes three points:

1. the youngster's craftiness in exploiting his mother's good nature has been learnt early;

2. good free writing (even if using a word processor) is heavily dependent on good spelling, because good spelling allows the wide oral vocabulary to be used actively in written form;

3. fostering spelling independence takes time, thought and tact.

Try this: Next time there's a story to write look at the clock as your child starts work and during the next five or ten minutes count the number of words you are called on to spell. Then say 'Since you started I've told you how to spell ten (or twelve or fifteen) words. For the rest I'll only tell you how to spell five words out of six (or four out of five) and the sixth one you'll have to work out by yourself. I won't even say yes or no, I won't nod or shake my head. At the end we'll proof-read' [184].

Give him a dictionary and see how the end of the story shapes. Is it grossly skimped? If so, next time record it first, as mentioned above. But if all goes well, after a while you can increase the number of words he has to write independently. Or, if he has a good picture dictionary, you could refuse to provide any words which are in it. Without fail, praise and reward honest efforts at spelling independence, focusing on the items he has got right. Say, for instance, 'You've got most of that word right, all your letters are right and in the right order, there's just one letter left out and it's a silent one'; don't say, 'That word's wrong, and that one and that one.'

If the above is too abrupt a withdrawal of spelling support, try this: He asks, 'How do you spell "collision"?' You write a continuous line and say:

'This line is for the word. Can you say it again and listen for any letter sound you can hear in it?'

'"Collision" – l.'

'Quite right. Where along this line do you think the "l" will come? At the start of the word, the middle, the end, nearer the start, nearer the end?'

He can write the 'L' on the spot along the line he thinks appropriate, or you can do it for him – including the doubling – or, if you are using a computer, the letter can be keyed in.

Now, working from the 'L' in position on the line, repeat the question, but this time, as the word is repeated, run a finger along the line so that it matches the 'L' as it is pronounced. Suppose the 'N' is identified next. Ask, 'Does it go before or after the "L"?' Insert as required, and continue, using letter sounds.

This technique, a kind of SLACAWAC in reverse [180], will involve you and him in articulating the word very clearly several times. All audible letters should be readily identifiable. You may have to jog his memory or supply spelling patterns that are unfamiliar, like the soft 'ce' in 'voice'. There will be opportunities for pointing out a small word inside a big one, a common letter string (like the 'tch' in 'kitchen'), a spelling rule, a prefix or a suffix that affects the meaning of the word.

Two more ideas recently reported at the clinic were enjoyed by the children: One mother admitted 'I can't spell either, so I got two dictionaries, a list of spelling rules and we're learning together. I need to spell for my Open University course.' It was working for the boy – we didn't test the mother.

Another mother found that she and her seven-year-old were jointly learning how to use the home microcomputer. A ten-word spelling program was the first they had successfully made. This had been so much enjoyed that two more programs, each of several groups of ten words, were planned, and mother saw herself prospectively tied to the micro watching her youngest whizz through the five levels of spelling lists used in his school.

Notice the shared fun element in both suggestions. It echoes the advice that goes out with all home-school reading schemes.

Proof-reading

184 The more tired the writer and the longer the written piece, the more difficult it is to proof-read it. Ideally the piece should be put aside for half an hour, or overnight. Children are in more of a hurry. Persuade your child to put aside the written piece, even if for no more than five minutes, during which his eyes will not engage with print or script. In this pause look at the written piece and see roughly how many misspellings there are altogether. Make up your mind how many you are going to ask him to correct. The number may depend on the school's spelling policy [179]. Call him back to his writing and announce the limits of the task: 'The target for today is correcting five (or six, or seven) mistakes. Can you find them?'

If he can find the required number and correct them, proceed to reward and praise. If he cannot find any, say to him, pointing to one line: 'In this line there's a misspelt word; can you see it?' If he still doesn't see the miscue, say: 'It's in the first (or second) half of the line,' and wait again. Only if he still cannot find the misspelt word, point it out to him and ask: 'What is this word?' He will probably say it correctly, but if not, let him read the whole sentence. Get him to say it with exaggerated spelling pronunciation, remind him of rhyming words, or break it up in a way that will clarify spelling: 'hap-pin-ess' (for the older child, 'happi-ness') 'in-con-sid-er-able' (for the older child, 'in-consider-able'). If it is a grammatically-based mistake, remind him of the rule, as with 'gradual-ly'. If it is a homonym confusion bring out a mnemonic, as in 'We can drive to our gran in one hour flat'. At first ask him to correct only a few miscues and gradually increase the number – though after a while they should decrease. But in general keep spelling work short (better to learn four words a day than sixteen in one fell swoop), praise him a lot, keep it fun, talk about it and keep in touch with his teachers. They may want to praise you too.

The latest research confirms earlier findings that spelling mistakes in short function words (like 'with', 'they', 'which', 'who') are the easiest to miss. So proof-reading must pay particular attention to the one hundred commonest words in print, most of which fall into this category. These words are often learnt on the wing, so to speak, just by being seen repeatedly. If not, they may be taught by being written very large on a blackboard; 'shadow writing' in the air with arm fully extended; written on the child's back for him to write on the blackboard [168]; with a thick felt-tip on the pages of an old telephone directory, finally scaled down into the exercise book. In short, they lend themselves to spelling through handwriting [183]. Equally difficult to spot are long content words that follow a specific phonological or grammatical rule – for instance, 'circular', 'longitude', 'emphatic', 'courageously', 'accredited', 'irregularity'. For these the answer, apart from

SLACAWAC [180], is to learn the spelling rules [172], analyse words [171], use a dictionary, and even learn some Latin.

Summary (180–84)

If your child has to learn 'spellings', help him.

Copying a word X times is seldom an effective means of memorizing it.

Proof-reading is a habit to be actively encouraged.

Word games and crosswords are enjoyable aids to spelling.

Assured cursive handwriting is a powerful prop to spelling.

Chapter Fourteen
Handwriting

Preamble

Handwriting is still a necessary skill and, despite increasingly sophisticated aids, looks like remaining one for the foreseeable future. Its
importance for schoolchildren lies also in its use as an aid to reading in
the early stages, and to spelling throughout. Getting handwriting to the
pitch of an easy, automatic skill takes a long time. Schools use a variety
of approaches, not all equally conducive to getting it right quickly. Like
all the other literacy and language skills described in this book, it starts
at home. It too is dependent on adequate vision and visual perception,
adequate control of eye movement, hand movement and the writing
tool.

Which hand?

Most of us 'write with the right hand'. If your child does too, it is easy
for him to tell left from right by remembering the pun. But he will be
trying his hand at writing, or at least drawing, long before he can
reliably name his left and right.

185

    In the reception class in Great Britain (or kindergarten in the
United States), that is, at the age of five, there will be some children who
have not developed hand dominance (a sustained preference for using
the right or the left hand). For them, writing will be that much harder.
The child with mixed hand dominance takes longer to establish the
habits that make writing comfortable: how to sit, where to place the
paper, how to hold the pencil, whether to write mainly by 'pushing' or
'pulling'. The right-handed person writes by pushing the hand away
from the body (whatever the individual strokes of particular letters
may do), leaving what they have written open for easy inspection. The
left-hander pulls his writing towards himself: his body can get in the
way of free arm movement and more often than not he covers with his
writing hand what he has just written. He has to be shown how to re-
position himself so that he can read his own writing to obtain immediate
feedback.

In short, for good practical reasons right-handedness is prefer-able. If you can channel your child into it without fuss it will make his life easier. On the other hand, it is definitely not worth having a long running argument over it. Whatever you do, don't encourage party tricks like writing with both hands equally fast. More elaborate versions are writing with both hands simultaneously in the same direction, or writing with the left producing mirror-writing. The last may have suited Leonardo da Vinci but is of no benefit to the child learning to write and spell.

Pencil hold

186 From the age of about fifteen months a toddler is capable of grabbing a pencil, especially a fat one, and scribbling. It is a satisfying experience for him. From the age of two and a bit, assuming his language is sufficiently advanced, he may also label his scribble 'dog', 'car', or whatever he can name and continue scribbling with increased pleasure. Having started by holding the pencil like a dagger, he may continue this hold till about three, or until he is shown how to hold it in the conven-tional three-finger grip. You could try showing him how to hold the pencil when he is about eighteen months and a few children get it right from the start. More commonly the dagger hold progresses to the spoon hold, with the thumb under the pencil and the fingers over it, the blunt end of the pencil sticking out beyond the little finger. The next stage is the flat hold, keeping the middle and index fingers on top and the soft thumb pad to the soft pads of both, the pencil still held not far short of upright. This sometimes slips, with index and middle finger curled over the pen, little and fourth fingers under and thumb protrud-ing. The conventional hold, with pen lying back, is often not learnt until school has started. Other things being equal [21], this early school-learnt skill should be mastered round about the age of five.

Triangular pencil grips encourage the bent index finger to rest lightly on the pen. The newest moulded-plastic pencil grip gives precise grooves for index, thumb and middle finger and leads to much im-proved writing. Triangular pencils from museum or cathedral shops do the same less well. The pencil tip should protrude no more than two centimetres beyond the fingers. The same grip is recommended for left-handers, but the tip can protrude by as much as 4 cm without loss of comfort or control. This higher grip will ensure that the writer can see immediately what he is writing, without having to lift his hand off the paper. This is important for feedback, especially in spelling.

Schools often have regulations about writing implements to be used. Generally, children are more likely to develop serviceable handwriting if they are allowed to choose from a wide variety the one that suits the individual exactly and so they overcome any incipient problem. A fountain-pen is held at an angle of about forty-five degrees to the paper and a fibre-tip or roller ball more upright, but the child's comfort is the guide here. Fibre-tips and roller ball pens move in all directions with equal ease and are therefore best for remedial exercises, should these become necessary. With these pens the variations in the thickness of stroke are due to pressure rather than direction of stroke (although direction affects pressure). Pencils are comfortable at any angle and are therefore the easiest writing tools to start with (as long as the lead is soft), leading quickly to the 'kinetic melody' mentioned by one writer.

So an easy as opposed to a tight grip is required; supple movement of fingers and wrist, and free arm movement, are also needed. Holding the arms down and shaking hands and wrists often loosens taut hand and wrist muscles; rotation of shoulders loosens arm movement. Both will be familiar to pianists and both are useful for the child who, after a spell of writing, complains, 'Oh, my hand hurts.' However, if the shoulders show signs of weakness, exercises to strengthen them will also stabilize the arms, easing writing and other fine motor activities.

While the standard pencil hold is the likeliest to lead to legible writing, children often vary it in the course of one piece of writing. With the young ones this may be because the standard grip has not yet become established. They need a brief rest, possibly a triangular pencil grip, and a reminder how to hold the pencil: for at this early stage the aim is to encourage the best handwriting processes until they become automatic. With older, more practised writers the variable hold allows easing of the muscles into a temporarily more comfortable position. As long as the variations of hold maintain legible, quick and comfortable writing (not hidden by the writing hand for left-handers), take no notice. Left-handers often hold the pencil in a very tight grip. They need the muscle-relaxing exercises described above; doodling and scribbling in continuous lines is also helpful.

Position

The business of handwriting will be more comfortable if the child sits square to the table. The height of the chair should allow his feet to be flat on the ground, the lower leg making a right angle to the floor, the thighs parallel to the floor, the trunk bent slightly forward and the

187

upper arms at not far short of a right angle to the writing surface. In short, no sprawling over the table; nor should the table be so high that the shoulders are uncomfortably raised. For shoulders and arms need to be easy if wrist and fingers are also to be easy and able to control the writing as required. At least half the forearm should rest on the table, to stabilize it. This too makes writing more comfortable and better controlled.

For right-handers, place the paper so that its bottom left-hand corner is about level with the right eye and then twist it slightly to the left. (Think of the line from six to eleven on a clock face.) Some right-handers prefer to keep the paper square to the table edge and have the forearm at a slight angle, as described. For left-handers, place the paper so that its bottom right-hand corner is about level with the left eye and twist it to the right, but it should be at more of an angle than the twist for right-handers. Many left-handers prefer to sit further from the table than right-handers, to give the left hand and arm greater freedom of movement. Depending on the development of the reference eye [44], younger children will arrange the paper more or less centrally or twist it at a greater or lesser angle. In every case the line of writing should be nearly parallel to the edge of the table, with the writing moving sideways away from the body for right-handers, and towards the body for left-handers. The paper should be held steady with the other hand.

If you notice that while writing your child lays his head on his arm, or supports the head with the non-writing hand, or tilts his head to look at the paper from various angles, or shifts in his seat, or moves his paper, always changing the angle of vision, don't complain that he is fidgeting. Instead, ask yourself if he is slow to read, finds spelling very hard, and handwriting a terrible strain. If the answer to any of these is yes, seek help from your doctor. He may refer you to an orthoptist to check the convergence of your child's eyes or perhaps his reference eye [44]. The doctor may ask what sort of light the child habitually writes in, or whether he has got used to writing with inadequate light, in partial shadow. This is only too easy when school working tables are crowded with books, collages, and all the usual bits and pieces of the classroom. Try to correct this at home: for right-handers light should come from the left and for left-handers from the right.

A habit to discourage

188 Some children, while sitting correctly square to the table, place their paper at such an angle that it lies across the body. Consequently for right-handers the writing is moving straight ahead and away from the face, or for left-handers directly inwards towards the face. What is written is then seen at an unconventional angle, with the individual letters sideways on. So the 'V', for instance looks to a right-hander like an arrowhead travelling from left to right.

When writing in this direction the child has to (a) hold in mind the meaning of the word he wants to write, the sound and the visual image of the whole word; (b) hold in mind the auditory and visual pattern of individual letters in sequence; (c) while holding in mind the visual sequence of letters, shift it through ninety degrees, and go on holding the auditory pattern steady, as well as the meaning and the visual image of the whole word (as in (a) above); and (d) write down the shifted visual pattern while holding the rest steady. This amounts to much more work than is normally necessary when writing a word from memory.

Assuming that the final version of the word, so laboriously achieved, is correct (a large assumption), the visual unit – the whole shape of the word – is still not like its twin on the conventionally placed paper. To see that e v e r y
is the same as

the child has to twist his head, or his body, or the sheet of paper. And he will certainly not find it any easier to remember how to spell 'every' because his memory of his own written version of the word will be significantly different from his memory of seeing it conventionally placed. So until your child is a very good reader and a reliable speller, please see that he positions the paper as described in the preceding paragraph.

Start writing

At last the child is sitting comfortably, with the paper placed to allow the forearm and hand unrestricted movement across the sheet. And he writes, preferably something that includes all the letters of the alphabet. Notice the movement of the hand at the wrist, from lying right on the outer edge of the little finger to something more nearly upright. The fingers are also moving, pushing the pencil in the upward strokes, pulling it for the downward ones. This is a lot more noticeable if the writing is large, and of course a child's handwriting starts by being large. For first practice in writing individual letters, the teacher

189

may well encourage her young pupils to trace the letters in grooved practice tablets. In these, the tall letters (like 'b', 'h', etc.) and the low letters ('g', 'j', 'p', etc.) are some fifteen centimetres from top to bottom, with the small letters (a', 'c', 'e', 'm', etc.) correspondingly proportioned.

Not that letters are necessarily the first and certainly not the only form of early writing: straight lines (horizontal, vertical, diagonal, crossed), shapes (circles, triangle, square, oval, lozenge/kite, double cross, figure of 8), continuous patterns (for instance arched loops and low loops) with many attractive elaborations each incorporating some of the movements needed for writing letters – all these are early forms of writing. If the child finds these difficult he will be encouraged to do them on a large scale, often on the blackboard, using the whole arm fully extended, with the 'writing' correspondingly very large. The aim is to achieve control of large-scale, gross movement and then refine it to control small-scale, fine movement. So if the fine movement is not up to standard (in practice, what the teacher thinks is reasonable in the first, reception class) the aim is to backtrack to the stage of development at which a particular movement can be executed with mastery, automatically [193].

For school purposes, absolute minimum ability is drawing on the blackboard, using one hand only, a horizontal line going from left to right, that is, stretching about halfway across the blackboard. (This is the beginning of handwriting – straight lines – as mentioned above.) At the age of five a child should be able to do this. If he cannot manage this movement of crossing the mid-body line (the central line down from the nose), watch him try. Does he start the line nearer the right-hand side of his body and then step sideways as he draws the line? Does he start with the left hand, get so far towards the centre and then change the chalk to the right hand to finish the line in the right-hand half of the blackboard? Or does he draw a section of the line, drop his arm, then start again just about where he left off? If any of these methods are still being used at the age of nearly six, consult your family doctor, lest it be part of a general delay in motor development.

Letter formation

190 With hand–eye coordination good, pencil grip secure and easy, and fluency of continuous writing movement well on the way thanks to practice with writing patterns, the method of letter formation remains open to debate. School policy has a lot do with it. Is the start made with capitals or lower-case letters (often called 'little' letters, to many children's confusion)? Are the handwritten lower-case letters to replicate the print in the first readers, or do they have small linking strokes at a very early stage? Is it to be h **or** h ? The formation of the following letters is particularly open to debate:

f b p   q j g   s x z

For handwriting, letters fall into four groups:

1. round ones, written anti-clockwise, and the hardest to form correctly:

a c d e g o q

2. line and loop, written anti-clockwise:

i j l t u y

and also, if rounded,

u w

3. line and arch, written clockwise:

b h k m n p r

4. the odd ones:

f   s x z

and also, if strictly diagonal,

v w

Visually, the letters most open to confusion are:

(very rarely)	f and t, y and h
(rarely)	w and m, n and u
(commonly)	b, d, p, q and g.

There is no need to worry if the confusion with the last group, and especially 'b' and 'd', persists until the eighth birthday.

The fine movement of handwriting can lessen confusion by:

1. writing 'f' so that it is a letter which both grows tall and drops low: f

2. writing 'h' with a small linking stroke; giving 'y' a hook to the left and not joining 'y' to the letter following: h y

3. writing 'v' and 'w' with high linking stroke: w

4. starting 'm' and 'n' with the straight downward stroke (to stabilize the shape and make joining possible), closely followed by the arch, or 'tunnel', as one young writer called it: ı ŗ n m

5. starting 'd' in the middle and forming it 'like an "a" growing tall', with a small linking stroke: ˧ c d d

6. starting 'b' at the top of the ascender (the tall stroke) and not joining it to the letter following: ı ↓ b

or starting 'b' at the top of the ascender and finishing it with a 'bow' (the 'script b'): ʖ

7. not joining 'p' to the letter following: p

8. giving 'g' a hook to the left and not joining it to the letter following: g

9. giving 'q' a small tail to the right and not joining it to the following 'u': q q u

Since practising individual letters can become boring, try 'discover and classify' games (particularly good with the lower-case alphabet):

1. Which are the tall letters?   b, d, h, k, l, t
2. Which are the low letters?   g, j, p. q, y
3. Which are the middling letters?   a, c, e, i, m, n, o, r, s, u. v, w, x, z
4. Which letters have a dot?   i, j
5. Which letters have to be closed?   a, d, g, o, q
6. Which letters do you start writing by going backwards for a tiny bit?   a, c, d, g, o, q, s, e, f
7. Which letters start with a low stroke?   p, j
8. Which letters have a high linking stroke?   σ r, v, w, and 'script b', ʖ, if used
9. Which letters are like half another letter?   r = $\frac{1}{2}$n, n = $\frac{1}{2}$m. Can he think of any others?
10. Which letters don't join the letters following (this is very much a matter of school policy, but these are the most commonly so used) b, g, j, p, q, s, y ('b' is omitted if 'script b', ʖ, is used)

11. Which letters have a bow? ┣ (watch out for school policy), capital R

12. Which capital or lower-case letters have a cross bar; A, G, H, J, T, f, t

13. Which capitals have two or more cross bars? E, F, Z

14. Which capitals have diagonals? K, M, N, R, X, V, W, Y

15. Which capitals are closed? B (twice), D, O, P, R, and even Q, unless the young writer argues that 'the tail opens it'.

16. Which capitals are the same as lower case? c C, s S, x X, z Z, and also p P, which serves to point the importance of position on the line.

All these help the child to focus on the details of the shapes of letters and the direction of letter formation, bringing the memory of the movement involved to help out visual discrimination of the differences. If at the same time the lower-case letters are identified by their sound, as in c = k, and the capitals by their name (H = aitch) the reinforcement loop through visual, kinetic and auditory channels is complete.

There is a brief but delightful period when the young writer thoroughly enjoys showing off his knowledge of letters to any indulgent adult or bemused younger sibling. At that stage he will both ask the questions above and provide the answers, demonstrating that for single letters he has now mastered formation and sound–symbol association.

Clarity and speed

As a child progresses through school, the amount of writing required of him increases and he has to continue reading back what he has written. So it is no longer enough to write (and often name or sound) each separate letter accurately. In word sequences the letters have to be distinguishable from one another, and the words must be separated by spaces. A gap 'as wide as your little finger' between words takes a while to become a habit.

If the child consistently and despite tuition writes letters so that they overlap and incline at quixotic angles, it is as well to check his vision and visual perception [65]. If at first the letters move up and down, on and off the line like a caterpillar, don't worry. A much commoner and more persistent source of confusion is that letters or parts of letters are incorrectly proportioned relative to each other. In school this is dealt with by exercise books with double lines to accommodate the 'middling' letters – 'a', 'c', 'e', etc. [190] but many reminders

191

are necessary before correct proportions in everyday, as opposed to 'best', handwriting become automatic. Until mastery has been achieved it may be desirable to remind him to check his piece of writing for 'tall tall letters' and 'low low letters'. Or you could turn it into a joke: a felt-tip of one colour can be used to go over the tall letters and another colour for the low ones. As long as he is not colour blind (fortunately very few girls are) this is an easy aid to correct proportion. You may find that only a few letters are misproportioned (the 's' is often too tall, even when fluently written), or only some letters in some combinations, for instance 'h' after 'w'. Once the commonest cause of confusion – or teacher anger – has been located, it can be specifically corrected. Don't insist on fine points, like capitals being taller than tall letters, or 'b', 'd' and 't' not being as tall as 'h', 'k' and 'l'. Calligraphy is a separate skill and pleasure, taken to very readily by children with access to word processors. But it can be lived without. What the child is after, as soon as possible, is legible cursive (that is a running hand), which involves joining up.

Cursive, or joined-up writing, is an aid to speed rather than clarity. Its introduction is very much subject to school policy: some junior schools don't like it at all, many delay it until the last year, others push it as soon as a child is ready for it. In the last case, in any one form small groups of children will be at different stages of learning how to join up. Whatever the policy of the school, there is no point in sacrificing legibility to speed, because the child's competence in reading (especially in the early stages), spelling and sentence construction will be dependent on the feedback obtained from his own writing.

Often left-handers retain legibility at the expense of some joining up. Do not expect your left-hander necessarily to join letters to 'a', 'c', 'd', 'g', 'o', 'q' and 's', the ones 'you start writing by going backwards for a tiny bit' [190]. These are the most difficult joins.

The easiest letters to join are the ones where a simple extension of the linking stroke upwards will lead to the starting-point of the following letters, for instance pairs of letters like 'ui', 'it', 'me' and 'ey'. The other important aid to legibility is to keep the distinguishing high link of 'o', 'r', 'v' and 'w' to the letter following. If the high join droops, as it so often does, 'o-s' looks like 'a-s', 'v-s' like 'u-s', and 'r-s' and 'w-s' like meaningless improvisations. The cross bar of the 'f' and 't' (and 'script b', if used) serves as a link to the following letter and as such is a guide to keeping the letters correctly proportioned. The 'f' is best distinguished if it is written as both a tall and a low letter.

The three commonest defects of established cursive writing are:

1. closed letters are not closed, so that 'a' looks like 'u', 'd' like 'cl', 'g' and 'q' like 'y'. There is nothing for it except to go over them again, or re-practise writing closed letters, which is boring,

2. moving the pencil with little flicks of the fingers rather than fluent movements, leading to strokes going in all directions,

3. distorting the low letters so that the descending strokes become almost horizontal under the writing line.

The cure for the last two is a return to writing patterns, with large flowing movements writing in the air, trying to re-establish kinetic melody.

There is one curious feature about the correction of handwriting: the teacher, or in extreme cases the occupational therapist, will persevere, demonstrating, guiding, trying to establish better habits, and at the end of the course she may seem to have achieved very little apart from guilt at her own inadequacy. But six months later a glance at the handwriting of the (as she thought) unsuccessfully treated pupil will reveal startling changes for the better. So it looks as if a long period is needed for digesting the better handwriting practices and putting them habitually into the required sequences. In short, mastery of serviceable handwriting takes a long time to acquire.

Why the fuss?

Parents may well question the amount of space and attention devoted to the details of handwriting. There are two reasons for this. Serviceable handwriting, as we have said, takes a long time and often much practice to acquire, and in the excitement, fun and urgent demands of junior schooling, acquiring this mastery is sometimes not given high priority; and handwriting, even under the guise of calligraphy, is seldom positively taught in comprehensive schools. In the authors' experience there are a considerable number of eleven- and twelve-year-olds whose skill with handwriting is just not up to the demands of secondary schooling. So here is an area where practice at home can make a significant contribution to performance, starting perhaps with a fresh look at choice of pen, paper position, quality of writing surface and the redesigning of the formation of some letters. In some handwriting programmes, usable at home, the exercises are graded with spelling in mind. Pairs or longer strings of letters which form common spelling patterns are practised, first just as joined letters and then as parts of words: 'ange' will be followed by 'strange', 'angel', 'dangerous'. Practice at home will therefore have double value, quite apart from the gain in

192

self-confidence from having worked independently through a series of graded exercises.

Secondly, though it should perhaps have been mentioned first, handwriting is the central skill essential in the early stages of reading, when beginners learn to read from what they write. The beginner builds up a personal data-base of words that he can write from memory with all the letters in correct sequence. If he fails to acquire this writing vocabulary despite reading from a distinctively illustrated reading scheme, the chances are that he is not distinguishing the visual differences of the printed words and as a result he cannot remember to read them in a different context. Handwriting is used to supplement his developing visual perception and correct any faults in it. At this early stage eye and hand work in close harness, each monitoring the other's performance and each providing a trigger to the memory.

Working on the principle that once a child knows how to write a word correctly he also knows how to read it, the child's reading vocabulary can be expanded through handwriting – and cheerfully at that. You need an old telephone directory and some thick felt-tips. Start off with a short word that he knows, for instance 'in'. Let him write 'in' in large letters, joined up, on several pages, each time with a different colour, until 'in' is written with mastery. Each time let him say the letter sounds and then the complete word. Expand this to 'win', again repeated in several colours. Alter the initial 'w' to 'b', then 'd' (careful that the two are formed in different ways, and the 'd' joined to the 'i'), 'f', 'g' (if gin is habitually in the house), 'p', 't' and 'sp'. You will find that, as the joke progresses, he speeds up in both writing and sounding. Next, tear out the pages and arrange them in a pattern, by colour, or height or depth of initial letter; use them to shape a snake, a fish, a car, but keep them all going in the one direction, so that he can re-read them consistently. Stand back and admire.

Clearly this sort of joke lends itself to considerable variation and any words that at later stages of junior school need to be learnt for 'spellings' [181] can be treated in the same way. This is one of the reasons why, in the common weekly task of learning to spell a number of words for a test, the words are very often grouped by similarities of spelling, or letter string. Consequently the task may include five words that end in '-ang' and five that start with 'dr-'. On the day of the test the teacher, instead of simply dictating the words, may give the definitions instead; so the child, on hearing: 'Write down the opposite of "wet"', has to remember the word 'dry', relate it to one of the two groups of words he has learnt and, knowing the initial 'd' and 'r', search his memory only for the remaining 'y'. The memory of how the fingers form and the eye checks the total configuration of the cursively written word 'dry' acts as the fly-wheel to enable the concept to be rendered on paper.

Parents faced with children complaining about the weekly 'spellings' chore may think all the above amounts to an exaggerated claim for the benefits of easy, legible handwriting. We think not. A few years ago, a series of children aged nine to eleven who came to our clinic complained loud and long about their problems with spelling and brushed aside any possible shortcomings in other aspects of class performance. The usual tests were done, the results collected and sent to the statisticians for impartial analysis. The doctor expected the children's performance on a test measuring their memory for sequences of abstract symbols to be the crucial ingredient in their ability to spell, or perhaps their performance IQ [69]. The teacher expected their accuracy of reading or knowledge of phonics to be decisive. The occupational therapist made no predictions but analysed the samples of handwriting. She turned out to be right: the sub-skill which was far and away the most closely related to spelling proficiency was legibility of cursive handwriting.

In short, efficient cursive handwriting is a necessary precondition for correct spelling of single words, but, according to the authors' most recent experience [173], not a sufficient one.

Approaching reading and spelling through handwriting works much better with children below the age of eight than with older ones, and for a short spell at that. If prolonged, boredom sets in. So it must be just one of a number of strategies designed to get a child reading and spelling. The reason for not relying on this approach exclusively or predominantly is that it works by conditioning to improve the memory. In this it resembles approaches devised for children with specific reading difficulties. The three best-known of these are the Gillingham–Stillman, Hickey and Fernald Multisensory approaches. The last has been subjected to precise research, which shows that it does lead to gains in literacy but only for children with difficulties in visual processing. In the authors' experience the improvement is again greater with younger children, and similarly the dangers are boredom and information overload. All three approaches emphasize auditory skills, leading to regular drill sessions of about half an hour every day. This is of little use to a child with a history of hearing impairment or to one who may be unable to generalize from the drilled examples. Further, the three approaches, and several other systems based on the same principles, give children only one strategy for coding and decoding messages: to rely on memory. The child's own thinking is not mobilized to tease out the message of the text. There is no scope for independent knowledge or judgement or skills in problem-solving and concept formation. Finally, all the systems mentioned above call for special training, special teachers, special materials, special teaching conditions and consequently special expense. Some people swear by them, but in general we do not.

Summary (185–92)

A child has to be shown how to sit, place his paper and hold his pencil for comfortable handwriting.

A child has to be shown how to write each letter with the correct movement, and has to practise letter formation.

From the start, legible handwriting is the main prop of early reading.

Joined-up writing also has to be taught and practised.

Legible, easy, joined-up writing is a great help to spelling.

Chapter Fifteen
Living and Learning

Preamble

This chapter is a ragbag of various points that have frequently cropped up in the twelve years of our clinic's operation. Each one of them has been explained to parents, children and teachers, and has proved useful. With luck they should prove useful again. Many will be familiar. The suggestions are offered without prejudice. You can but try them.

Stages of learning

In acquiring any skill or competence with a task, whether it is spelling, or dressing, or making scrambled eggs, the learner goes through three **193** stages.

Stage one, when the skill/task is broken down into its constituent sub-skills and these are practised separately – in the case of spelling, the sub-skills would concern word meaning, letter sound, phonic pattern, syllabication, likely letter string, derivation, grammatical rules, sentence structure, overall shape, etc.

In *stage two*, these sub-skills are practised together in whatever the appropriate sequence might be: pulling up shorts, getting head and arms through the correct openings of jersey, pulling on socks, putting on shoes, doing up buttons and belts, tying up shoelaces, and so on.

In *stage three*, full command of sub-skills in fluent sequence has been achieved. The sub-skills are used rapidly and automatically, the sequence varied as necessary, with the user often unaware which sub-skill he's using at any particular moment.

For instance, if a child aged seven, who has been shown how, still finds it impossible to write the figure 8 in one movement, the teacher or occupational therapist may have:

1. ascertained that he knew the terms: up, down, left, right, across;
2. made sure that he had a serviceable pencil hold;
3. written the figure very large on the floor and asked the child to walk over it;

4. asked the child to finger-write the 8, as large as possible, in sand, with his hand guided as necessary;

5. asked the child to finger-write it on a sand-paper board, possibly saying a guiding mnemonic while he does it;

6. written a very large figure 8 on the blackboard and guided the child's hand while he traces over it in coloured chalks, still using the audible mnemonic;

7. asked the child to trace over the figure 8 by himself, but still with the audible mnemonic;

8. asked the child to write the figure 8 from memory, first with and then without the audible mnemonic;

9. asked the child to write the figure from memory while chatting to the teacher or therapist.

The last stage amounts to mastery of writing a large figure 8 on a blackboard. It still has to be transferred to paper and the scale reduced. Obviously there is, in practice, a considerable overlap between the stages. For instance, a nine-year-old does not need to know the meaning or be able to spell words like 'vociferously', 'disengagement', 'encapsulate'. But he does need to have the skills that enable him to break the words into syllables and have a shot at getting his tongue round them.

Styles of learning

194 Not all children learn in the same way. Some are very hesitant. They start from what they know for sure – that 2 red and 2 blue bricks make 4 bricks altogether – and move in tiny, often-repeated steps to the next point of certainty: that 2 red and 3 blue bricks make 5 altogether, or that 3 red and 2 blue, or 4 red and 1 blue, or vice versa, make 5 bricks, and they remain 5 bricks on the floor, on the table, in the sandpit, on the window sill. It takes a very long time, but the information taken in is well and truly accepted.

Some children are more resolute. Give them a puzzle, say a pattern with a 'bite' taken out of it and a choice of six pieces with which to finish it. They will pick out the missing piece very quickly, but then, assailed by doubt, they will try all the other pieces too, just to check they've got it right. These children also believe in belt and braces. Bolder spirits will plump for any old answer and then gradually refine it to the correct one. The tearaway will pick out an *ad hoc* answer – never mind if it is correct or not – and immediately move on to the next excitement. The reflective ones will consider silently all the possibilities, give a considered reply and stick with it.

These responses can be graded along a continuum running from the pedantic to the careless. A child learns faster and more thoroughly if the learning experiences are presented to him in the style that he favours. In practice, this applies particularly at the two extremes. The very uncertain child needs tiny tasks, where the possibility of failure is just about eliminated. In spelling, for instance, he will feel happy with exercises where changing the first letter of a word gives him a fresh one signalled by a picture: 'hat', 'mat', 'rat', 'bat'. The tearaway will only be persuaded into careful spelling if he has a crossword which hides the clue to the treasure in his current Fighting Fantasy book.

You know your child. If you are trying to 'bring him on' with puzzles, games and exercises at home, remember to find the ones that suit his learning style. Make sure the belt-and-braces chap has time to check out all the possibilities. In the long run it saves time.

Early learning skills

Research done in Canada and repeated in the United Kingdom shows **195** that a child who is a good reader at the age of eight is likely to have entered school, aged five, able to do the following:

1. show by his answers that he is paying attention;
2. settle down well to an activity that needs some concentration;
3. cope with something new without getting nervous and upset;
4. fall in with the general activities of the class;
5. try on his own;
6. accept help when he cannot manage some task;
7. be alert and interested.

Just common-sense, you will say. Quite so. The use of common-sense hallowed by research is in leading the teacher to precise observation of her pupils. If the seven abilities listed above always apply to your child, all well and good.

If they apply only sometimes, the teacher should identify the occasions when they do not: at the end of the day, just before lunch, in the hay fever season? She also has to decide on the precise form and severity of his non-fulfilment of the seven criteria. A second questionnaire, divided under fourteen headings and three levels of severity, is then used. By considering your child with these guidelines in mind, the teacher has to define what she finds worrying or unacceptable. She can then tell you specifically where she sees the trouble as lying, perhaps that 'he rushes in without taking time to look and work things out'. Is he often unobservant, answering without thinking? Does he guess cheerfully unless positively reminded to take time to think? Or does he never stop to look or think out an answer?

Don't be offended if the teacher talks about your child in this way. Credit her with intelligence, good-will and expertise different from your own. So think over what she has described. Does your child behave in a similar way at home, and if so, to what degree, in what circumstances? Then discuss the matter again with her. Between you, work out a way of guiding him into more reflective behaviour without damping his imagination and high spirits.

If the early learning skills are very poor all round, and the teacher decides to call on outside advice, the questionnaire above, or a similar one, could be the basis of discussion between her, you and the outside adviser. In that case ask for a copy of the questionnaire, with the teacher's ticks, crosses and comments. Again proceed quietly, for there is no benefit whatsoever in quarrelling with teachers, schools or education authorities. They are as anxious for your child's successful schooling as you are.

Talking

Purpose

196 To labour the point: if at any stage a child's oral language is not up to standard his learning will suffer, and learning includes reading, writing and spelling. Starting young, a child must understand what is said and then reply. Equally, he must be able to start conversations in response to experience, as a means of making sense of it and of keeping in touch with other people. The earliest stages of this process have been described in the sections on language. As a child gets older his reasons for contributing to conversation become clearer, because his utterances fall into broadly recognizable categories:

1. making demands/commanding: 'Give me (more often "gimme") that';

2. reporting experience: 'There's pussy getting over the fence';

3. commenting on other people's experience: 'Mike got his cornflakes on the floor.'

4. collaborative intention/instruction (and this marks a big step in the social development of the child): 'I'll put it here and you hold it like that.'

5. role play/pretend games: 'I'm the ticket man and I say, "Any more fares please?"'

6. asking questions, seemingly for ever, but always needing patient answers, in the hope of fostering the reasonable approach to life;

7. boasting ('self-maintaining' is the jargon for it): 'I'm a very strong boy.'

The older child
With the older child, experience, not least of reading and writing, will influence the way he talks.

197

1. Demands are mellowed into requests (sometimes, in the case of the older teenager, formal ones) and persuasion (including arguments to support or demolish a point of view); or made on behalf of a group, possibly as a means of negotiating for the group.

2. Reporting from personal experience is to cover descriptions (including descriptions of emotions); re-telling of past events, including later, the self-denigrating funny anecdote; re-stating something recently learnt. This may take the form of exploratory talk, thinking aloud in order to clarify meaning, and may be part of group discussion. All will be heightened by analysis and comparison with other, similar personal experiences.

3. Commenting on other people's experiences expands to take in comparison with the speaker's own experience in a similar field; expression of the speaker's emotional response and perhaps identification with the person being spoken of; judgement, that is, various degrees of support or criticism.

4. Collaborative intent will extend to description of an activity or task to be undertaken, the reasons for it and prognosis of its likely future course; pinpointing contributions from collaborators, discussion for joint construction of an idea and re-formulating knowledge ('making knowledge' is the jargon for it); the speaker will monitor his own and his collaborators' action, support some speakers and deal as necessary with controversy or direct challenge.

5. Role-play is transformed into telling original stories; re-telling someone else's story but with an original ending and suggesting possible alternative courses of events; dramatizing some recent experience, preferably one shared with the peer group. This would again lead to identification with other points of view.

6. Asking questions continues vigorously and calls for an open mind to absorb and express various arguments and hypotheses, with more exploratory talk to sharpen the outlines of a problem and plan

solutions; explanation of processes, which may call for evidence of precise observation; recognizing general principles, as, for instance, talking in order to clarify mathematical concepts.

All the above are self-maintaining in the sense that they serve to add to or shape the child's social, intellectual and moral abilities.

As the child becomes conversationally more adept, he will consciously alter the way he speaks in response to a particular situation and his relationship to the person he is talking to. This should spill over into the way he writes. Generally the first distinction that is noticed is between narrative and transactional prose, for instance the language of a fairy-tale and that describing the rain cycle.

He will be able to contribute more fruitfully to classroom discussion – and with luck improve the construction of his essays – when he recognizes the routine often followed in teacher-orchestrated talk for learning.

1. The likely start is a broad question, for example: 'Why were the Crusades undertaken?' Major contributions to the discussion are wanted, based on some factual knowledge and imaginative thinking.

2. The next step is the shepherding of pupils to a full response by (a) following through their ideas with first evaluations of their importance; (b) focusing on particular facets of their answers; (c) checking for inconsistencies, contradictions or irrelevant points.

3. The teacher may then suggest that extra relevant information should be sought; comments on these additions are intended to keep pupils thinking on the subject, to draw out inferences and extrapolations.

4. Main ideas will be summarized, to show what conclusion may be drawn, or what further questions need to be asked.

Telling a story from pictures

198 One of the most reliable ways of getting children to talk is to encourage them to tell stories while following a sequence of pictures. These are commercially available, starting with three and going on to a maximum of seven. Some have two cards for the final episode, to allow for different interpretations leading to alternative endings. This is the method:

1. Choose a sequence of cards and arrange them in the right order. Present the first to the child and, after a pause for him to consider it, ask: 'What do you think is going on here? What do you

think has happened?' The aim is to guide the child into understanding and putting into words the main message of the picture. Later the same will be required in reading, when the main idea contained in a paragraph has to be identified.

2. Ask some follow-up questions, to get at the supporting details. The same search for supporting detail will later be needed using information from text.

3. The next set of questions should elicit the reasoning behind the incident on the card: 'Why are they having a picnic?' 'Why is the boy holding the candle?'

4. Entering into particular characters is then called for. 'What is the bus driver thinking?' 'What is mother saying to the boy?' 'What is the girl looking at?'

5. Finally, prediction: 'What will the man in the hat do next?' 'How will the fireman get the cat down?'

Showing the pictures one by one and asking the same type of question with each should not only get the child thinking about the pictures and increasing his scant conversation by talking about them, but should also nudge him into understanding how the different elements of a story are carried forward from one episode to the next, to build up the narrative.

Another version of the same activity is to give the child all the cards of a sequence, ask him to arrange them as he wishes and then ask the same types of question. More practised story-tellers can make up stories on the basis of paired 'why/because' cards, or just one picture. This can be specifically designed to encourage conversation on a particular topic (such as seaside holidays); alternatively a photograph or a reproduction can be used. If the picture includes a person or an animal looking out of it at the story-teller, more questions relating to the characters can be asked. These often lead to the first realization, for the child, that the story-teller or reader actively participates with the author in the re-creation of a story.

Story-telling and re-telling

Story-telling flourishes in a happy, relaxed atmosphere with the parent visibly attending. Even if you are ironing or sewing, stop every now and then, look at the teller and put in a comment or a question which signals your absorption in the tale. The more interested the audience, the greater the self-confidence of the story-teller.

Your child's stories will start by being personal narrative, a mix-

199

ture of fact and fiction, the parts connected by 'and', but even these are a preliminary stage of his ability to generalize his experience. Later, his stories will give him the opportunity of hypothesizing – the 'supposing' gambit – and of using the past, present and future. Verb tenses give him more precise wording for the passage of time measured by a sequence of events.

Your child will also be hearing stories and will start re-telling them. This will give him familiarity with story-telling conventions, which in turn will ease his own reading of stories. He may also re-work a story he has heard, which is another way of recognizing experience. The more he re-tells real-life anecdotes or heard stories the more fluent he should become, because, with the content familiar, he can concentrate on the style of story-telling. If encouraged to tell and re-tell, he will go on getting better at story-telling.

In short, personal and heard stories are, for the younger child, a most important way of organizing his understanding of the world, of expressing his own ideas, and of thinking about himself in his expanding world.

Games

200 All children play more or less elaborate pretend games. They are an essential part of growing up, they mirror the child's extending experience, and they stretch imagination, understanding and language. They should be encouraged and supported with props like dressing-up boxes (reception classes sometimes have racks of dressing-up clothes), and parents, if invited, should join in. All familiar ground, easy to follow and fun.

You, on the other hand, want them to play a game with a mildly educational purpose. Children are generally aware of this but cooperate willingly if the game is sufficiently enjoyable (and that means it should not be too difficult), if it anchors your attention on them and if a good atmosphere of shared fun is built up. It is wise to decide in advance what, apart from entertainment, your chosen game is meant to do. Is it to accustom them to the conventions of board games: taking turns, counters, dice, counting moves, penalty/progress cards? (Any number of games will do for this.) Is it to teach them something about the geography of Europe? (You will need a particular board game.) Is it to make them aware of fine differences in pictorial or abstract design? (There are a number of games on either the Lotto or domino principle.) Is it to speed up the ability to read common words, or to build up words from roots with prefixes and suffixes, or to group words into families? (A considerable range is sold by educational publishers.) Is the purpose to improve his ability to categorize? The 'Happy Families' principle has been extended to bilingual cards (French and English) to cover a wide range, from animals to orders of architecture.

If you are looking for activities as well as games to back up reading and spelling generally, there are many pamphlets that list suggestions and give examples. Ideally they should be small and transportable (some of the best, published by Harcourt Brace, are called 'Hip-Pocket Games' and the pamphlets literally fit into a hip pocket), so that the games can be played anywhere at any time. If you think your child has a specific problem and you would like to help him informally, time and difficulty may be saved if his problem is defined by a teacher or a developmental or diagnostic clinic. Precise suggestions can be made by a speech or occupational therapist. Some commercially available games intended, for instance, to develop visual perception may be held in the occupational therapy department and shown to you before you decide whether to buy them or not. Your child's teacher may consult a specialist adviser, who often holds stocks of special teaching materials to be loaned out as necessary.

You may like to consult the catalogues of educational publishers. Not all of them will sell to private individuals or, if they do, extend their trade discount to them. Your local book- or toy-shop may help by ordering for you. A local play-group or Parent–Teacher Association may also have a use for the particular game, so that once your child has grown out of it you are likely to find other takers for it.

All the above applies also to computer games, daily more numerous, absorbing and sometimes literate. For example, 'Macbeth – the computer adventure', from Oxford Digital Enterprises, is not only accompanied by the text which has to be combed for clues as an integral part of the adventure, but the clever player can twist the plot so that Macbeth survives. This is excellent for the reluctant reader being put through the English literature O-level.

On long car journeys, don't try to play games with educational intent. There are plenty of others, listed in booklets available at filling stations on the motorways. For a long, undisturbed spell, you could ask the children how many TV jingles and advertisements they can remember.

Travelling, holidays, outings and maps

Children come to our clinic from all quarters: the two most distantly based were from Karachi and Trinidad. You'd think a good conversa-

201

tion opener is to ask: 'How did you come here?' But many children of ten or even older have no idea at which station – main-line or tube – they boarded or got off the train, whether they came by bus or car, or whether they crossed Westminster Bridge or any other. With younger children it is common to have no idea where they live or where their school is. They are no better at knowing where they went for a much-enjoyed holiday. These children travel like parcels.

This is a slot that parents can fill very helpfully. 'Making the child aware of its surroundings' is the phrase that covers this large topic. The aim is, by using talk, to make the experience explicit and to tie it in with earlier experience or information; returning conversationally to the particular event will help to fix it in the long-term memory and be used to trigger anticipation of further similar experiences. Suppose you have taken your children on a day's guided tour of Pompeii. At the end of that dusty hoof your children will have seen and discussed things which tie in with their previous experience of:

1. Roman remains in England, and what they discovered about the Romans when 'doing' them in school, with any books – including the Asterix comics – about Romans and any TV programmes about them;

2. volcanoes, and what they learnt about them in school or saw on TV;

3. the organization of guided tours, including a meal in a restaurant.

When they return to school and are faced with reading material on any of the above subjects, your children will bring to it 'experiential comprehension'; this will enable them to predict sensibly what ideas, phrases and words are likely to come next, and they will in consequence make a much better job of reading and understanding the text. This is no more than an extension of the point made earlier [90] that language grows out of experience and serves to clarify, consolidate, enhance and anticipate it. So, roughly, the wider the range of experience and the more thorough its conversational processing, the better for language, thinking and reading development.

Holidays and outings are also occasions for tackling maps, which are very troublesome for a large number of children. The reasons are obscure [74], but if the case is not severe parents can do a great deal to overcome this embarrassing disability. Before going on holiday you might show him on a map where you will start and finish, and what route you propose to follow. If you are travelling by rail or car your

child can probably consult the map every now and then. At stops on
the way he can write in a little notebook the name of the stopping-
place, the hour of arrival, the distance covered since the last stop, what
the weather is like, the purpose of the stop. Has he seen anything
special since the last stop? A car crash, a satellite transmission station, a
travelling circus, a castle?

When you get to the end of the journey it is a good idea to chat
again. Is the place like home or different? Has he been there before, or
somewhere like it? Does it look like the brochure? Is there anything
particularly striking about it? Tourist offices often provide sketch maps,
with the main features of the locality in small photo inserts. What does
the sketch map leave out and why? If you are buying picture postcards
of the place, you might walk (following the map) to some of the places
on them and decide where the photo was taken. (With an older child
who is interested in photography a second theme of conversation develops at this point.) Could you relate the tourist map to the Ordnance
Survey or local equivalent? How far are you from home, grandparents'
home, a place he has been to or heard of? Can he, by reading the map,
suggest where he would like to go for a swim, a scramble over rocks,
fishing, photographing some special local event like hang-gliding, car-
racing, welly-throwing? Are there posters announcing events of this
kind in the area? The tourist map should indicate how to get to them
on foot or by public transport, car or mule. By involving your children
in planning some of your holiday activities you will be providing opportunities for purposeful conversation, again contributing to their
language development as well as their competence with maps.

History

Every school in Great Britain teaches history in one guise or another. It
infiltrates the junior school curriculum through 'projects' and later
either becomes a subject in its own right or part of 'humanities'. In the
last two years of compulsory schooling it is often part of a group of
subjects. If your girl chooses for her options – that is, subjects in
addition to the compulsory English and maths – to do art, French,
biology and dressmaking, she may find that she has to take history
also.

History more than any other subject is the one where, as adults,
it is hard to distinguish between what was learnt at school and what
was picked up casually in the normal course of travelling, reading,
viewing, visiting sites or exhibitions. From school days onwards the
informed response of the eye is as important as the knowledge of facts

202

and the habit of going back to sources. What can you do to foster, without fuss, an awareness of the past into which information can, at intervals, be slotted?

One of the best options is visiting historical sites. Depending on the age of the child, the choice varies in its usefulness to you as a parent. Even the most obstreperous six-year-old is hard put to it to damage a prehistoric, Iron Age or Roman site. They all lend themselves to story-telling, they are in the open air, often on top of a steep hill, ideal for exhausting exercise or breaking long car journeys. Medieval sites are trickier: castles are excellent and lead very rapidly to consulting books, but cathedrals do not encourage running about and to the unpractised eye are much of a muchness. With luck there is a memorable detail: the door-knocker at Durham, the map in Hereford, the green and white stripes in Siena. With children up to the age of thirteen or so there is genuine difficulty in sorting and remembering sites in periods. Could you help them by 'bringing in another modality', as the jargon has it, in this case taste? Your children may be clamouring for ice-cream. There are much the same ice-creams throughout Great Britain and several West European countries. Code the sites by ice-cream: raspberry ripple for Roman, flake for medieval, nut cornet for the eighteenth century, etc. It works.

Teachers, or a glimpse at homework, will reveal which period or theme is being studied at any particular time. There may be, within easy reach, related sites; the library may have picture-books, or stories to be read to and with him, to make the period more memorable. Historical books for children are numerous and generally of a very high standard.

For older children preparing for public examinations, a particular period or theme will be set. Could you visit the relevant sites at home or on the continent? Is there an appropriate exhibition, a room in the local museum which relates to the period being covered? It's probably wiser not to be deflected from the period being studied, so if you are concerned with the eighteenth century, resist temptation to have a quick look at the Great Bed of Ware. Is there a book of the 'they were there' type? Eye-witness accounts of the Gordon Riots, or of Fanny Burney being chased by poor old George III are as evocative as any TV programme. You could discuss the issues raised by large-scale technological changes: was building the network of canals round Birmingham as disturbing for the local inhabitants at the time of the industrial revolution as the siting of nuclear power stations is in ours? How do the responses compare? These historical explorations can be a focus for relationship between parents and their teenage children. The chances are that all will be starting on an equal footing, discovering the past together, adding equally to the store of information and self-awareness. It can be a very good interlude in what are, sometimes, strained relations.

Reading for maths

The young child gets his first ideas of space and proportion by moving in space. The more chairs he crawls under, the more sofas he climbs over, the better. It is tiresome for you when he unpacks the kitchen cupboard or a bookshelf, but it's good for his perception of space and proportion. At the earliest opportunity he might be guided into another useful activity: does he unpack your vegetable basket when you bring it home from the shops, sorting potatoes, onions and carrots into their separate containers; does he pick out the number of spoons needed for two, three or four children's ice-cream; later, does he lay the table, counting the requisite number of spoons and forks? Cooking at as early an age as possible is a good mathematical aid: could he help weigh out the ingredients for a cake? 'Put in currants until the needle points to the 4 here', and he'll be reading the dial and recognizing the digits very early. When the ingredients are mixed he might help spoon the mixture into paper cases and arrange them in neat rows on the baking-sheet. Suppose he also adds a cherry to each (and eats one or two on the way), he will soon realize that three rows of four little cakes, or four rows of three, add up to twelve. When you make biscuits, how about letting him stamp them out and arrange them in rows or clusters on the baking-trays? If you have a vegetable garden, does he help you peg out the spaced rows along which he then evenly trickles the seeds? Does he make a scale plan of which vegetables grow where? An older child could help you work out how many tiles are needed for a floor, or how much material for curtains.

From talking with him you will realize how well he understands concepts of time, distance and height, but is he sure of the unit of measurement? Can he express his ideas of size, weight and distance in relation to a familiar object ('It's as long as my shoe') or in relation to conventional units?

If sums are brought home for 'finishing' or extra drill, an abacus or Cuisenaire rods are useful, and the book that comes with the latter is good. Many schools allow calculators, certainly in the run-up to public examinations. There are many good computer programs for 'drill and practice', but there is no point in getting a program about fractions if

203

he needs one to 'develop and reinforce addition and subtraction' [211, 212]. Booklets suggesting mathematical games are readily available, but they may contain the other booby trap in maths: the language of the books and workcards. Mathematical English contains a great many mathematical symbols, as well as graphs, charts and diagrams, which need a different reading approach from continuous prose in ordinary English. They use very compressed as well as necessarily very precise language, especially when giving instructions. (The same applies to verbal reasoning tests, done in the last year of junior school and one of the determinants of secondary school placement.) In mathematical English every word is important, in contrast to normal reading matter which contains redundancy so that the reader does not need to concentrate on every word in turn. Does the child know what is meant by 'plot a graph'? Does he know how to use a worked example? Does he realize that reading a maths book requires active reasoning with pen and paper to hand?

Individual schools, or local authorities, sometimes lay on a maths course for parents, to show them what is being asked of their children. In six London primary schools parents are asked to help their children practise maths at home. Enjoyment of the activities and the children's progress in class are monitored.

Computers

Preamble

204 Computers are now an integral part of education and easy familiarity with them is essential for life in the twenty-first century. Therefore, your child needs experience of computers, the earlier the better. Learning to communicate with a computer should be a natural process, giving the child early mastery over technology and extending his thinking power as soon as possible.

Given the computer is not a toy but a learning tool, the choice of hardware becomes important. Choose a micro that can be used as a word processor with a spelling checker, ideally with a printer as an integral part of the package. At worst it should be possible to add the printer with the minimum of fuss. Also, the micro should have a very wide range of programs available for it. So consult the makers' catalogues, the computer magazines (alas, since 1986, many of these, together with the smaller software producers, have bitten the dust), look for reviews in educational magazines, enquire at the local computer club, Parent–Teacher Association, College of Further Education, or the

Government sponsored Micro Electronics Support Unit or the few remaining LEA sponsored Micro Electronics Education Development Units.

Provision in schools

Will school provide the necessary experience? At the time of writing the answer is: yes and no. Schools are constrained by finance, although a vigorous Parent–Teacher Association, with enthusiasts among both parents and teachers, can make a very big difference. Schools are affected more subtly, but more thoroughly, by the attitudes of the local education authority, the head teachers and the staff. And a school will be limited in its freedom to manoeuvre and innovate in the computer field by the pool of skills and expertise available among the staff and, let's face it, by the scruples staff may have about infringing copyright by the illicit copying of programs. How much time does the timetable allow for computer studies? In junior schools, have topics that cross subject boundaries been chosen with a view to making use of suitable programs? Does the member of staff responsible for computer studies have a good or bad attendance record? Consequently, the extent of computer experience your child obtains may vary considerably from one school to the next. This holds true even if schools are geographically close and take pupils from closely comparable catchment areas.

Therefore you, the parent, may legitimately think that your child is not getting enough computer experience, as measured either by time spent at the machine or by the range of programs on offer. Before you express disappointment to the staff, make detailed enquiries about the amount of hardware actively in use, the type and number of programs at any one age/actively level, the number of hours per week or term allowed to each child by the timetable and how much extra time and experience may be had by joining a computer club based at school but taking place out of school hours. You may be dissatisfied by the answers and ask next what you could do at home to supplement school provision. Do not be surprised by an attempt to deflect you into making a significant contribution to the school's computer hard- or software instead. The unspoken argument against other forms of parental involvement is that parents will buy commercially available programs labelled as 'educational' by the makers, but will have no means of judging the educational value of such programs; they will therefore buy rubbish, which will do more harm than good. Even if, by some happy accident, parents may buy something of genuine value, the child will become familiar with the program, or the process that it teaches, and will therefore often be unwilling to use the same program in a somewhat different way in school; or he will be a clever dick and offer his own suggestions, at variance with the teacher's, about how a particular task should be tackled, or indeed subverted, for purposes of vulgar entertainment.

The official argument advanced against parents supplementing public education with computer programs at home will run something like this: use of a computer by a small group is a wonderful exercise in collaborative learning: a computer changes the social climate and therefore a mixed ability group can engage fruitfully, each child bringing his personal experience to a joint endeavour; with computers there are far fewer distinctly yes/no, correct/incorrect situations, so blame is not seen to attach to anybody and work in progress can easily be altered; while engaged in problem-solving, as thinking grapples with the task, language is generated through discussion and this collaboration leads to a great development of social skills.

All the above arguments are perfectly true and valid and valuable. The considerable amount of language generated is in itself an excellent development. However, parents may also have a suspicion that collaborative learning can go on at home as well as in school, that there may even be virtue in other aspects of computer use. They may also remember – or the child's grandparents may remember – the time when teachers asserted loud and clear that parents were not to teach their children to read, only teachers being capable of this task.

Provision at home

206 If you are wavering about whether to buy a personal computer or not, the answer is, get it. What will your child gain?

In the first place, plain familiarity with the machine. While all micros, like all sewing machines, work on the same principles, the more elaborate micros, like the more elaborate sewing machines, will perform a greater variety of functions by taking a wider variety of programs, which in turn handle a larger body of information. If your child has frequent access to the micro he will get used to operating it, and should therefore get beyond the stage where pressing the wrong key leads to elementary mistakes that take a long time to put right, or at least he'll get better at correcting them quickly. Secondly, since a computer is an aid to thought and you are trying to encourage your child to think his own thoughts rather than re-hash someone else's, you can supply programs which are open-ended. These programs are content-free structures into which your child builds what he chooses to. With these his learning, while entirely informal, will be self-directed, therefore active and probably predominantly private. This independent and personal aspect of computer-assisted learning is the opposite of what computers in schools are designed to achieve.

Programs

LOGO

The question remains, which programs to choose?

The first and absolutely essential one is LOGO. There are various versions of this on the market; the newest (at the time of writing) is very fast, in colour, and available for the cheapest computer on the market. LOGO, in its infant and junior-school versions, is associated with a programmable moving object, the 'Turtle', to which the child issues commands via the micro. In this way his pleasure in giving commands is drawn on to help him relate keyboard instructions to actual physical movement. The next level of sophistication is the screen Turtle, graphics on a VDU, immediately more complicated because the movements occur on a different plane from that of the physical movement of the child. The obvious importance of LOGO is for the child's understanding of direction, number, angle – in short, geometry. But the main reason for choosing LOGO first is that it gives immediate access to programming; from the word go the child teaches the computer to think and to remember, and incidentally watches himself thinking. So he can notice the differences between computer thinking, which is analytical, and logical, and human intuitive thinking. He will gradually realize that these two ways can and should be alternatively used and, later, in what circumstances either style is the more apt. The computer will nudge him into formulating his intuitive thinking, which, once it is explicit in the analytical terms of a program, becomes accessible to second thoughts, to examination of any one part of a given problem. So the computer is allowing the child to upgrade his qualitative thinking. Second, third and subsequent thoughts can be fitted in while he explores the micro-world of geometry (that is, maths stripped down to basics) in a series of genuine self-selected experiences.

WORD PROCESSING

Word-processing programs are another tool for upgrading the quality of thought. There are many on the market, with or without a 'dictionary'. This is a memory for so many words against which the user's own spelling of these words can be checked. However, the real value of a good word-processing program is that the child's own free writing is liberated from the chore of handwriting, with all the slow troubles of letter formation, letter size, rubbing or crossing out, and so drearily on and on. Words can be made to appear at speed, then reconsidered at leisure, and the flow of intuitive thought can be caught and held until the child is ready for the analytical process of editing. This will consist of the rearrangement of phrases, the re-wording of particular ideas and altering their order, additions (perhaps to include some fresh information), deletions, and the correction of spelling and punctuation. At each step it will be possible, painlessly, to return to the original and, just as painlessly, buff up some corner of it.

For the child who has difficulty in controlling handwriting the attractions of word-processing are obvious. The child whose memory for spelling is poor also benefits, because he can gradually check his way into correct spelling. The child who is incoherent on paper can produce sensible messages by sorting out his originally scrambled text. The child who writes too little can start by writing his usual scant minimum and gradually expand it. In every case the child's baseline is an acceptable and legible start. He is released from worry about producing a conventionally correct final text of desired quality, so he can concentrate on content. He can think – or talk, if this is being done collaboratively – his way through successive drafts, and see the value of having them. As long as he maintains the urge to communicate, he can only do better. Fortunately in practice computers extend the child's attention span and enthusiasm for writing beyond all expectations.

Both teachers and parents who have watched children using this type of program report the same results: an enormous improvement in content, a considerable one in length and variety of syntactic structure, and much greater willingness to take trouble with layout, paragraphing, spelling and punctuation. Handwriting becomes a separate skill, an art form.

Long-established, habitual use of a word processor for all written work should, if supported by letters from head teacher and doctor/psychologist, lead to use of the same in examinations like GCSE [214].

DATA BASE

209 The third content-free program that your child needs is one for information-handling. The child is free to collect information on a topic, organize it into a data base and store it on tape or disk. He can then interrogate the data base to extract specific items of information and to analyse it in a variety of ways. From the analyses he can make further deductions which in turn will suggest other ways of storing information on a fresh topic. This type of program, one designed to classify, is very popular with boys following the fortunes of a particular football team or athlete. Spread-sheet programs, for the older and more practised micro user, take this process to a higher level of sophistication. Confident use of such a program is something of a status symbol for the teenager. Parents are more likely to be impressed by the thinking that has to preceed the organization of information into the data base.

SIMULATIONS
Finally, there is the vexed question of simulations. These range from noisy space invaders to complicated exercises used in the higher reaches of university education: for instance how, in a given time and on a given budget, to eradicate malaria from an imaginary landscape – drain the stagnant waters, spray with insecticide, dose the population with prophylactics, or any combination of the three and in what proportions; what to do if the rainfall increases or decreases, and so on. The first is a solo exercise that improves coordination and brings no other benefit to the player, the second engages thinking processes of the highest order, sharpened in a collaborative exercise. The first is little more than a way of killing time, the second calls for decision-making, linking cause to effect, and, possibly, reference to other sources of information. Simulations to be educationally useful have first to be rational and then complex; the more complex the better, because the complexity allows for greater creative choice.

210

Consider a progression from snakes and ladders, to noughts and crosses, to Monopoly. The control and choice the player is exercising increases with each. Move on to the Business Game, Diplomacy or chess, and the element of choice in personal decision-making, and the thinking required to make it, is going to increase the sensation of personal involvement. So as a general rule the deeper the involvement of the players in the simulation the better, both for educational development and for fun.

Simulations can be based on well-documented experience, like flying a glider, which will demonstrate how air currents behave and how weather conditions, both local and general, affect them. This should lead to a consideration of the secondary issues involved: the provision of gliding clubs, the cost of equipment and its maintenance, insurance, safety precautions, recovery procedures, choice of sites, interference with low altitude flying, etc.

Alternatively, simulations can be on a fantasy theme, like *Dungeons and Dragons*, which takes the interactive principle still further and involves players in role-playing. These games are fun, including the planning and calculations involved. If the simulation is tied to a particular scource, like *The Hobbit*, the players may be led to the book, and with luck even progress to *The Lord of the Rings*.

In general, simulations are for children aged nine or more. There are, however, some very good simulation programs for use with younger children in schools and these are tied in with specific and closely defined teaching objectives.

DIRECT TEACHING PROGRAMS

What to look for

211 Frequently parents seek programs of direct educational value, 'something that will help Johnnie', usually with sums or spelling. They are looking for drill and practice programs, in the hope that the novelty of the computer will encourage Johnnie to buckle down when the same exercise on paper has left him cold; or that, in the privacy of the home, Johnnie will be able to learn at his own pace and not mind making mistakes before he 'gets it'.

When selecting specific programs, there are two groups of pitfalls to avoid. The first are technical. What programs will run on what micro? How long does it take to load? Will it crash? Is it legible? Does it wobble? Are the instructions clear? Seeking information on these points calls for objective judgement. It does no more than clear the decks, ensuring success with the contents of a program. It is the sort of information we no longer ask when we refer to books because the book, as a usable product, has been taken for granted for a considerable number of years.

The second lot of booby traps to look out for are the educational ones. Treat with caution all reviews in computing magazines. Ask yourself, is the review aimed at teachers, parents or children? Does it carry the endorsement of one or more local education authorities, teachers working in a particular institute or school, tutorial establishment or summer school, or coaching privately? If parents have watched the program being used at home by another child, was parental help needed frequently, occasionally, or not at all? Best of all, get hold of the names and addresses of earlier users and ask them what precisely the program aims to do and how well the aim was achieved, after how many repetitions, with a child or group of what age.

This is particularly important for programs sold as aids for dyslexics. As you realize, there are different kinds of dyslexia with correspondingly different teaching approaches and materials. The full range of materials has to cover all the levels of severity of the particular dyslexia. Therefore the programs will vary in both difficulty and kind. There is no point in overburdening a child who has trouble learning with an irrelevant program or a relevant one that is too easy or too difficult.

Far too often drill-and-practice programs offer the novelty of the computer as a means of holding the child's attention. They do little that cannot be done with paper and pencil. Your child may enjoy the graphics and sound effects so much that he persists in making mistakes for the electronically provided entertainment.

How to fit in with school

There is a further complication. Schools teach particular items in a particular order, or in a particular way. Take the example of spelling. While there are obvious landmarks that all spelling tuition roughly follows, the details can vary greatly from school to school. Your child may attend a school where five, or twelve, or twenty weekly 'spellings' have to be learnt and are conscientiously tested. Regardless of the merits of teaching spelling in this way, suppose you decide to improve your child's spelling competence by getting him a program that teaches the spelling of some four hundred words. 'Spell "ski",' intones the voice from the machine, and your child presses the appropriate key. Fine, so he knows how to spell 'ski'. But if you live in Florida or Queensland or Cornwall where snow is a three days' wonder and skiing a pursuit carried out in distant regions, what is the point of learning to spell 'ski' (particularly since it contradicts one of the basic spelling rules for English)? Are you overburdening your child's already shaky memory for spelling (otherwise why would you bother with the program in the first place?) with irrelevant information? Would he not be better employed learning how to spell 'swamp', or 'cove', or 'reef'? So before you start buying drill-and-practice programs find out how they fit in with your child's requirements. If there isn't a program that plugs the identified hole and you are a dab hand at programming, consult his teacher and invent a tailor-made one for him.

While you are consulting your child's teacher, ask how far the commercial program gives practice with a skill she expects him to have mastered already, to be mastering now, or which he will be asked to master next term or next year. This last point needs caution in another direction. Suppose your child is a mathematical prodigy, fully ready at the age of eleven to tackle and delight in quadratic equations. Do you get him programs that explore this area, and how do you know which

212

are the good ones? The teacher, when consulted, will be thinking of her class organization, amongst other things. If she has scope to keep your prodigy usefully occupied while the rest of the class are working their way through the normal curriculum, all well and good. But if she hasn't, if she is committed to teaching the whole class at the same level, she may try to dissuade you. Her dissuasion will be the more earnest if your prodigy's behaviour in class leaves something to be desired. You as the parent may decide that it is still desirable to support your child's interests. Good for you – but don't necessarily expect any thanks from the teacher or any advice on the quality of programs.

Sources of information

213 Information about programs should be sought from users, as mentioned in paragraph 204, and either individual parents and teachers, or particular organizations. For instance, the Independent Schools Information Service can provide addresses of preparatory schools that use a very entertaining and colourful series for teaching Latin. *The Times Educational Supplement* regularly carries reviews. So does the news letter from:

Advisory Unit for Computer Based Education
Hatfield Polytechnic Computer Centre
Endymion Road
Hatfield
Herts.

which also sells software directly to the public.
A different service is offered by:

Special Education Micro Electronic Research Centre
Newcastle Polytechnic
Coach House Lane Campus
Newcastle-upon-Tyne
NE7 7TW

Write to them, giving the make of your micro and a description of the disability; the Centre will, in return for a fee, search its Bardsoft Software Data Base and send you the print out.
If you are in the happy but disconcerting position of having a lot of apparently ill-sorted software, get hold of Metropolis, a system for effective software use from:

Computer Applications to Special Education
Department of Psychology
University of Keele
Keele
Staffs. ST5 5BG

Summary (204–13)
A home computer can be put to very good educational use.

Content-free programs (LOGO, word-processing and data base) are the most fruitful and give immediate experience of programming.

Simulations should be chosen for their rationality and complexity.

The quality of commercially available programs labelled 'educational' varies enormously.

Consult other users and publications about which direct teaching program to buy, and when and how to use it.

Keep in touch with school about what you are providing at home.

Public examinations

Public examinations are usually taken with an eye, often parental, on the future. Academic success at school determines what happens next. Any examination poses problems for the child with learning disabilities: he may have difficulty in reading exam questions; he may have problems in composing a decent answer; his handwriting may be illegible; his spelling unacceptable.

214

Examinations in the United Kingdom are controlled by a variety of organizations, depending on the type of qualification required. The commonest school examinations are controlled by six groups for the new GCSE. They will consider provision for any disability: physical, visual, auditory or specific learning difficulties. Since candidates are unlikely to fall precisely into one of those clusters, each case is considered on its merits. The child's head teacher should first consider which syllabus to follow and whether options allowing 100 per cent course work (done in the pupil's own time) are appropriate. If sitting an exam is planned, the child's head teacher should contact the examining group as early as possible, ideally very soon after the start of the two year lead into the exam. Very thorough documentation as to the exact nature of the child's difficulty should be provided. An educational psychologist's report is often required, as well as information from the physician as to the medical cause of the difficulty. Technology provides alleviating conditions: if a child has a long-established and medically accounted for difficulty with handwriting and has habitually used a word processor and printer for the bulk of his written work in secondary school, a letter from the head teacher to this effect should lead to the use of the word processor in the exam. At the time of writing more controversial, but gaining ground, is easement of the difficulty with spelling. If this has a medically-backed well documented and long-established history, the use of a word processor with a dictionary is likely to be allowed. Try to find out whether your LEA has a booklet setting out examination provision for candidates with difficulties and consult it as early as possible. If not, write to the relevant board for direct information. You should also remember that:

1. Granting an allowance may result in a Board issuing a special certificate which states that an allowance has been necessary. Not all employers or colleges regard these qualified certificates as the equivalents of ordinary ones.

2. Passing one level of an examination does not mean that the next level will be achieved. A pass is just a pass, not the guarantee of further success. It may represent a child's academic ceiling.

3. A job may bring interest, self-esteem and money. Another two years at the books may not.

Should you be seeking help?

215 If you have skimmed through this book with a particular child in mind, you may now be asking yourself: 'Should I be seeking help for Johnnie? I don't like to worry the doctor and teachers hate mums who fuss, but I'm still not happy about his progress.' What should you do?

Take a large piece of paper, date it and divide it into four. Head the sections *health, behaviour, social* and *learning*. Now, in the light of what you have read in this book, think about Johnnie and make brief notes in each section. Obviously some of the notes will overlap from one section to the next. For instance, is 'Always rude to granny' *behaviour* or *social*? But 'Prefers to play with younger children' is definitely *social*. By the time you have finished you may not think you have enough evidence to 'worry the doctor'. In particular you may have least information about Johnnie's learning.

The next step is to have a chat with his teachers. You may not like to express unease openly, but if there is a convenient open day or parents' evening the teachers' opinion can be obtained without drawing particular attention to yourself and Johnnie. You need to find out from the teachers how Johnnie responds to teaching over a period of time and how he fits in with his peer group and adults in school. As the teachers answer your inquiries they will be keeping three things in mind: the demands of the *curriculum* (which compares with *learning* above); the *social* context in which learning takes place, and the relationships in class and out that Johnnie has established (which compares with *social* and *behaviour* above); his *health* and how this affects his learning. When you get home, make notes of the teachers' comments under these three headings. Now compare the two sheets. To what extent do the observations of the teachers tie in with your own? Even if the teachers did not appear overly concerned, have they noticed the same traits as you have? Does Johnnie prefer to play with younger children in school, as he does at home? Consider whether the two lots of observation add up to a consistent pattern. Do you and his teachers attach the same weight to your joint observations, or are you alone in your worries?

Suppose you decide that your worries are now without foundation. You decide not to get in touch with the doctor, at least not for the time being. But don't throw the two sheets of notes away. Keep them for three to six months, even a year. Look at them again. Have things altered? Take a fresh piece of paper, date it, divide it into four and write the headings: *health*, *behaviour*, *social* and *learning*, as before. Again, think of Johnnie under these headings. Has he stopped being rude to granny; is he rude or aggressive with a wider range of people? Is he silent and withdrawn, or is he friendly and outgoing occasionally, frequently, or not at all? And with whom? Is learning in school going better, or more slowly, and is he cheerful about going to school? How many heavy colds has he had since you last made notes? Has he had an illness with a high temperature, a fit, or an accident? Has there been a new baby in the family? Has Johnnie acquired a new skill, like swimming the length of the pool? If you have another opportunity of talking to his teachers, make notes on what they tell you under the same headings as before.

Compare the two sets of sheets. Do they seem to you to be describing a good or a bad trend? Or do they describe a situation that is static but, because of lack of development over a period of time, unsatisfactory? Or is Johnnie's progress steady but so slow that he is falling ever further behind his peers? Do you want to talk to his teachers again, or do you want to go straight to your doctor? Or will you leave it for another three months? If you decide on the last, repeat the noting of observations at the end of your self-imposed time interval. And if then, after considering all three sets of notes, you decide to seek further help, take all your records of structured observation with you to the doctor, the psychologist, or the adviser who is to be consulted.

Reasons for orderly note-taking

216 If you record your observations into ordered notes you will, for a start, yourself get a much clearer picture of Johnnie's functioning and development. It will be easier to disentangle the main features from the details of the worrying – for you – aspects of the situation. For instance, you will see which kinds of behaviour are present always, which frequently and which rarely. You will be able to discover whether some kinds of behaviour have become more frequent or more marked, or less so, or whether your tolerance threshold has altered. You are also likely to be reminded of various triggers that precipitate worrying behaviour. For example, if there is a standing fight over homework, does this happen every time, or just on days when a particular subject is set, or occasionally when there is a particularly pressing club meeting? If a new type of worrying behaviour has started, by remembering the time when it did so you may be able to relate it to its exact trigger, perhaps an illness or an accident. Secondly, if you are seeking help for Johnnie you will have to describe the trouble and how you react to it. Your structured notes will enable you to make a much better job of this essential communication. Thirdly, the doctor will find it easier to grasp the features of the situation if he is helped out by a record of structured observation, especially if the record stretches over a period of time. A doctor, backed by a multidisciplinary team carrying out a variety of tests and examinations, will obtain something akin to an enormously detailed still from a film. Parents' and teachers' reports provide the moving picture, the dynamic setting into which the still fits. Both are needed if your child is to get the help he needs and deserves.

Chapter Sixteen
The Law

The 1981 Education Acts in the United Kingdom
Provision for children with special educational needs is governed by the
Education Act 1981, and in Scotland by the Education (Scotland) Act
1980 amended by the Education (Scotland) Act 1981. These Acts are
based on the Warnock report of 1978, which recommended that:

217

1. services should be planned on the assumption that one in six
children at any one time, and up to one in five children at some time in
their school career, would need some form of special education;
2. categorization of pupils by handicap (for instance 'partially
sighted', 'educationally subnormal') should be dropped and the focus
should be on the needs of the individual child;
3. children with long-term/severe/complex disabilities should be
(a) assessed by a multidisciplinary team, and (b) recorded as being in
need of services not generally available in regular schools.

In other words, a spectrum of learning difficulty is seen to lead to
a variety of special educational needs requiring a spectrum of provision.
The 1981 Act defines a child with special educational needs as:

1. having a significantly greater learning difficulty than the
majority of children of his age;
2. having a disability which either prevents or hinders him from
making use of educational opportunities generally provided for children
of his age. A mother tongue different from the language of instruction
is not, by itself, a learning difficulty within the meaning of the Act.

Duties of local education authorities – the 'statement' child
Each local education authority has the overall duty to provide special
education (that is, education additional to or different from what is
regularly available for children of a particular age) for pupils with
special needs, and to keep the arrangements for this, in respect of every
individual child, under review.

218

Consequently the LEAs have, in detail, the following duties:

1. to identify children with severe/complex/long-term difficulties, whose special needs will require special provision;

2. to assess the needs of each of these children on the basis of a multiprofessional assessment and draw up a statement of needs and provision;

3. to educate each 'statement' child in regular school as long as (a) parental views are taken into account; (b) the efficient education of the other children in regular school is not adversely affected; and (c) educational resources are efficiently used.

4. To review the progress and needs of every 'statement' child at least every twelve months;

5. to re-assess the 'statement' child between his fourteenth and fifteenth birthdays.

The 'statement' child – assessment

219 What follows is an outline of the steps taken before a child is provided for by means of some form of special education. The details of the steps will vary from one local education authority to the next. Parents are advised at the first whiff of 'statement' to find out what the administrative steps in their authority are, how far the process has gone, and the names of the people concerned. The educational psychologist is generally the linch-pin of the evolving arrangements.

The head teacher, or teacher with pastoral responsibility, may think that a child on the school roll has special educational needs of a scope that would warrant a full assessment leading possibly to a 'statement'. He should start by discussing this informally with the parents, educational psychologist and possibly the school doctor, covering especially what the child's needs are and what has so far been done for him. If there is agreement that 'statement' status might be desirable, the next step is a formal request, on a form, and generally through the educational psychologist, for a full assessment. Parents are at liberty to refuse, but they must be formally notified of the LEA's intention to proceed to a full assessment.

Equally, parents are at liberty to initiate proceedings; they can lodge a request with the LEA for a full assessment under the terms of the Act. An unexpectedly large number of parents try to have their child 'statemented', because, once a child has been 'statemented', help for him becomes the statutory responsibility of the LEA. Head teachers realize that a few 'statemented' children on the school roll will lead to regular provision of an additional and specially skilled teacher. LEAs are torn between the demands of the parents under the Act and the perennial shortage of funds. Whether parent or LEA first raises the possibility of 'statementing', it is the educational psychologist for the school who formally initiates assessment procedure. Once formal assessment procedures have been started, parents have twenty-nine days in which to submit written evidence and/or make representations to the LEA. Further discussion is in order before the LEA sends (as it must, by law) to the parents a copy of the proposed statement. On receipt, parents have fifteen days in which to meet an officer of the authority, or any of the assessing professionals, and make further representations. Therefore more discussion is possible before the LEA, having considered these further representations, either stays with its statement (that is, the proposed statement becomes the substantive one), or makes a revised statement, or makes none at all. In any event the LEA must:

    1. inform the parents which of the three above courses of action is being followed;

    2. send them a copy of the substantive statement;

    3. give them the name of a member of the LEA from whom more information and advice about the child's needs can be obtained;

    4. inform them of their right to appeal to an appeals committee.

So far, appeals have rarely been necessary since the proceedings leading to assessment and preparation of the statement offer an opportunity for the resolution of differences. The appeals committees are expected to include members with relevant knowledge of special education, who will have the parents' statement and representations available. If additional information from a professional is requested from the LEA or further evidence is provided by the parents both must be made available to all parties. Parents have a further right of appeal to the Secretary of State.

In the authors' experience the period from request for statement to statutory provision, varies from six weeks for the thwarted murderer to two years for the well-behaved child with a specific learning difficulty.

Provision at the coal face

While, as Warnock says, twenty per cent of the school population will have at some time some special educational need (and the authors support this figure), only a small proportion of them will qualify for

220

'statement' status. Therefore provision for the whole twenty per cent will be graded – with variations for the individual LEAs – roughly as follows:

1. regular teacher provides extra help in the regular classroom;
2. regular teacher, with help from other members of the regular school staff and school-based resources, provides extra help either in the classroom, or another room on the school premises;
3. regular teacher provides extra help with materials brought in from a resource centre;
4. the child is seen by an outside, visiting specialist teacher/adviser who prescribes further tuition and perhaps supplies specifically targeted material or selects suitable materials from the school store;
5. part-time attendance at a special class;
6. full-time attendance at a special class;
7. full-time attendance at a special school.

Warnock envisages the following children as requiring special schools:

> . . . those with severe or complex physical, sensory or intellectual disabilities who require special facilities, teaching methods or expertise that it would be impracticable to provide in ordinary schools; those with severe emotional or behavioural disorders who have very great difficulty in forming relationships with others or whose behaviour is so extreme or unpredictable that it causes severe disruption in an ordinary school or inhibits the educational progress of other children; those with less severe disabilities, often in combination, who, despite special help, do not perform well in an ordinary school and are more likely to thrive in the more intimate communal and educational setting of a special school.

There is a wide range of possibilities by way of helping a child with special needs before the 'statement' procedure is even thought of, so do not be alarmed if your child's school suggests that he should be seen by a specialist teacher/adviser/educational psychologist. These are professionals whose job it is to obtain the best service for your child, largely by advising his regular class or subject teachers. In secondary schools some children may need extra support with the curriculum; others may need the curriculum modified to suit their special educational needs.

For optimum development children need to be grouped in a variety of ways for their different learning experiences; indeed, a greater diversity of learning experience needs to be thought out and offered to them. This is recognized by the LEAs who are the first to appreciate the basic complication of special needs provision: the differences between children with learning difficulties are far greater than between children whose learning goes smoothly and rapidly.

For children below school age, the evidence for special needs is collated by the district health authority through its nominated medical and nursing officers.

In Great Britain the first port of call for worried parents should always be the family doctor. Information from school will also be needed. The doctor may refer the child to a hospital or other specialist centre, while the school may seek help from the educational psychologist or specialist adviser on the staff of the local education authority (address in the telephone directory). Independent schools have similar advisers on call. Write to the Independent Schools Information Service (ISIS), 26 Caxton Street, London SW1.

Employment and the learning-disabled

A child with a learning disability may have been designated as having 'special educational needs' under the 1981 Education Act. This will have meant that he was unable to take advantage of normal schooling and therefore had to have special help which the educational authority had to supply. *Children who have no problem other than an inability to speak English, because it is not their mother tongue, are not classified as having 'special educational needs' within the meaning of the Act. Such children may of course have a learning disability, in which case they qualify for special help.*

Once the child has left school, the Education Act no longer applies and therefore the special education ceases, though there may still be a need for it. Help must be sought from Adult Literacy classes, which are provided by many different agencies. Start by asking at your local Citizen's Advice Bureau.

The youngster may have either a learning disability making him functionally illiterate (i.e. with a reading age less than that of a normal ten-year-old), or a physical disability such as partial deafness, or a combination of both. He may have considerable difficulty in finding employment, even with the assistance of the local Careers Officer.

A small study carried out in south London illustrated the extent of the problem. Over a hundred firms each employing more than a

221

hundred people were asked two questions: (a) did they employ people who could not read English (for whatever reason), and (b) if illiterates were not employed, how were they, in the first place identified?

Half the firms employed up to five illiterates and most firms used a job application form as a means of identifying them.

It is possible to estimate the 'readability', that is, the reading age necessary for comprehension, of any text. Most of the firms were asking for a reading age of twelve and some for one of fifteen or over. The jobs on offer included those of cleaners, machine operators and canteen staff; very little reading was required for the efficient performance of their work.

If the school-leaver's reading disability has persisted in spite of special help, then it may be worth his while considering registration as a disabled person. Nobody likes to be thought of as disabled, least of all a physically fit youngster who is a whizz at football. But some laws are there for the benefit of the individual and it is worth looking at what the law has to offer. Under the 1944 Disabled Persons (Employment) Act, employers with more than twenty workers have a duty to employ a quota of registered disabled persons. At present this stands at three per cent of the total staff; car park attendants and passenger electric lift attendants do not count towards the quota as their jobs are specifically reserved for the registered disabled.

The Companies Act 1980 contains the Companies (Directors Report) (Employment of Disabled Persons) Regulations which apply to most companies employing more than 250 people. (For the purist, a Regulation does not have the legal force of an Act, but does carry some weight in law.) The companies are required to make a statement in their annual report describing the policy applied during the previous financial year for giving full and fair consideration to job applications from disabled people, having regard to the applicant's particular aptitudes and abilities. There is also a need to describe the policy for the training, career development and promotion of disabled employees.

The Manpower Services Commission has formulated a 'Code of Good Practice on the Employment of Disabled People' and a publication is obtainable from H.M. Stationery Office.

One caveat: employers may see the functionally illiterate as being at risk under the Health and Safety at Work Act. In section 2, this Act requires that it shall be the duty of every employer to ensure, as far as is reasonably practicable, the health, safety and welfare at work of all his employees. It is possible for that to be used as an excuse not to employ illiterates or semi-literates 'because they will not be able to read safety notices'.

THE LAW

Before considering registering as disabled, the school-leaver should discuss the pros and cons of such action with the people in the Disablement Advisory Service at the local Job Centre. They will be in touch with the local Careers Officer and will know the position with regard to local firms.

If the question of the Health and Safety at Work Act arises, the Employment Medical Adviser (you can find him under the local Health and Safety Executive in the telephone directory) should be consulted. He should be able to say whether there is any real risk attached to a particular job in a specific firm. He works both for the Manpower Services Commission and for the Health and Safety Executive and can get in touch with the School Medical Service if necessary.

In short, do not reject the question of registering as a disabled person. Leave no stone unturned in order to get a satisfactory job.

Republic of Ireland

The national educational policy with regard to children with special educational needs is to enrol them in ordinary classes in ordinary schools. This is possible to a very substantial degree because the majority of such children are handicapped only by experiencing more than usual difficulty in mastering literacy and numeracy. These children are supported by remedial teachers supernumerary to the usual teacher–pupil ratio; these teachers have had additional training with literacy and numeracy over and above what is compulsory for all primary school teachers. Remedial teachers either teach small groups withdrawn from regular classes and do this on the school premises, or act as devisers and providers of teaching materials, or they team-teach alongside class teachers, either in the regular classroom or in special classes attached to some primary schools.

A number of children with visual and hearing impairment are also enrolled in ordinary schools. They are supported by teachers trained to deal specifically with these handicaps. These highly specialized teachers also act as advisers to other less highly qualified teachers and to the families of the handicapped children. Physically handicapped children can increasingly attend ordinary schools because, following special building guidelines, access to school premises has been greatly eased.

At post-primary level, handicapped children may attend special classes that have been set up at some second-level schools throughout the country; alternatively they may attend a special school. Ireland being a thinly populated country, specialized schooling of high quality can be provided for many children only in a residential setting. But a

222

scheme of home visits enables pupils to keep in close touch with their families. Children in special classes and special schools have their progress reviewed annually by a multiprofessional team. They will in the first place have been referred to the special school only after an assessment by such a multiprofessional team, on the basis of psychological, medical and educational reports.

Regional Health Boards (through their Directors of Community Care) and the Department of Education cooperate in providing ancillary support and home tuition for children who cannot attend school regularly. The National Rehabilitation Board provides a youth employment service for young disabled school-leavers.

ADDRESSES
Department of Education
Marlborough Street
Dublin 1

National Association of Teachers in Special Education,
c/o St John of God School
Islandbridge
Dublin 8

Association of Remedial Teachers of Ireland
c/o Teachers' Centre
Drumcondra
Dublin 9

New Zealand

223 Education in New Zealand is compulsory between the ages of six and fifteen. It is centrally funded and provided, free and secular, by the Department of Education, under its permanent Director General of Education. An elected minister is answerable to Parliament. There are a substantial number of independent schools, mostly denominational. The Department of Education checks standards in both state and independent schools. Primary and intermediate schools are administered by local education boards, secondary schools by boards of governors. The general policy is to educate as many pupils as possible in ordinary schools, especially in ordinary classes in their local primary schools. The local education boards employ itinerant teachers to help children with a hearing handicap or serious reading difficulty, who are nevertheless integrated into ordinary classes. Reading and speech clinics are also administered by the local education boards.

Handicapped pre-school children can attend part-time groups attached to selected kindergartens and play centres.

Once in a primary school, handicapped children are integrated in the regular class whenever they can, individually, benefit from the arrangement. Some primary and intermediate schools have special classes or resource centres attached to them. For instance, in the Auckland District (one of ten covering the whole country) there are sixty-one special classes at forty-seven primary and intermediate schools. At selected secondary schools there are special classes for the deaf, the backward or the maladjusted. When necessary, buildings are modified, special equipment provided and ancillary staff appointed to help the regular class teacher. Further help, especially in devising suitable teaching programmes, is available from specialist advisers, Department of Education inspectors and psychologists. The last are members of the Psychological Service, which offers a comprehensive diagnostic and advisory service for children with learning or social difficulties. They also liaise closely with all secondary school guidance staff and the health and welfare services for children.

The other specialized guidance services are:

1. the Hearing Assessment and Guidance service, which offers guidance to parents and teachers of the deaf;
2. the Visiting Teacher service, whose members liaise between teachers and parents of children whose school progress is held back by home difficulties;
3. advisers on handicapped children, who advise parents of handicapped children and the children themselves.

The Department of Education administers the state special schools, which are mostly small day schools with twelve to a hundred pupils. There are seven residential ones, two for the deaf, three for the backward and two for the maladjusted. Special classes in hospitals and psychiatric hospitals are administered by local education boards.

Looked at from Great Britain, educational provision in New Zealand has two remarkable features. The first is the multiplicity and excellence of its speech clinics (a service provided directly by the Department of Education), 148 of them, divided into ten districts, each under a District Speech Therapist, and attending to nearly twice as many children as receive full-time special education. The second is the success of two practical approaches to literacy: Marie Clay's on reading and

Arvidson's on spelling. Any teacher of English reading and spelling is indebted to them.

ADDRESSES
Education Department
Regional Office
Gillies Avenue
Newmarket
Auckland

Education Department
Regional Office
P.O. Box 12345
Rossmore House
Molesworth Street
Thorndon
Wellington

Education Department
Regional Office
123 Victoria Street
Christchurch

Mr J. S. Taylor
Secretary
Association of Independent and Integrated Secondary Schools of
New Zealand
Rathkeale College
Masterton

United States of America

224 Provision for disabled children operates at three levels: the federal, the state and the local education area (school district). At the federal level the important development was the 1975 Education for All Handicapped Children Act (also known as PL 94-142 – PL standing for Public Law). Even while it was being passed, the lack of money to implement it was obvious to all concerned and voiced by President Ford. So to keep expenditure within manageable limits, 'All Handicapped Children' was interpreted as enjoining the fifty states of the Union to provide specialized education for children with all types of impairment and to limit the number of handicapped children to twelve per cent of the entire school population between the ages of five and seventeen. At the time of writing one quarter of the handicapped children, three per cent of the entire school population, are deemed to be learning-disabled.

Since each individual state provides its own educational services, PL 94-142 laid down conditions for parting with federal funds. To qualify, a state must fulfil the following conditions:

1. It must locate, identify and evaluate every handicapped child within its jurisdiction.
2. The evaluation must be non-discriminatory.
3. Children must be placed in the least restrictive environment consistent with their needs.
4. Parents or guardians must be given fundamental due process rights.
5. States must pay for all educational services and guarantee all rights to handicapped children in private schools or facilities, as well as those in publicly-funded schools.

PL 94-142 defines a disabled child as:

1. having one or more specifically listed disability (he must be mentally retarded, hard of hearing, deaf, deaf-blind, speech-impaired, other health-impaired, multi-handicapped, or have learning disabilities);
2. requiring special education, educational tools and related services.

At the school district level there is, as enjoined by the law, a tendency towards 'mainstreaming' – keeping as many handicapped children as possible in the regular classroom. The regular class teacher may call on support personnel within the school, and/or an itinerant teacher who is a specialist. The teacher and the child can make use of the resource room. If the severity of the handicaps is beyond these 'in house' aids, part-time attendance at a special class may be sought, or even full-time attendance. Another degree of severity calls for a 'home-bound programme', the next for a special day school, and the last for a residential programme. All these provide a spectrum of services. Generally a number of school districts, each providing one or more components of the spectrum, combine their several special education resources to operate in concert.

The school districts have the mandatory duty to provide individualized education programmes (IEPs), one for each child. These documents must contain information about:

1. the child's level of educational performance;
2. annual goals;
3. short-term objectives for achieving the identified goals;
4. special education and related services to be provided;
5. the extent to which the child will be able to participate in the regular education programme;
6. projected dates for starting and the anticipated duration of services to be made available;
7. objective criteria, evaluation procedures and schedules for determining, at least annually, whether short-term objectives are being achieved.

As the IEP is being compiled, parents are of course consulted and, where possible, the child also.

There are two more nationwide services for handicapped children in the United States.

The Development Disability Services help nine per cent of all physically and mentally handicapped people. Autism, epilepsy and cerebral palsy come within their remit. The services concern themselves with identification, treatment (medical, dental, prosthetic devices, etc.), residential services, developmental education (for example, self-care, mobility, speech), transport, leisure activities and counselling.

The Crippled Children's Services also concern themselves with locating children who may need medical care, but the focus is on those who are physically disabled. They provide health care for the child and financial assistance for the family, rehabilitate the severely handicapped, and encourage early diagnosis and treatment, and high standards in medical care.

Across the United States there are 125 established categories of handicap, but some states have more extensive coverage than others. As well as shifts in their definitions of eligibility, state provisions vary widely, mostly keeping in step with the strength and vigour of parental groups lobbying for legislative action.

ADDRESSES
Association for Children and Adults with Learning Disabilities
4156 Library Road
Pittsburgh PA 15234

(A pressure group with 800 branches, its members are parents of children with learning disabilities and interested professionals. The stated aim is 'to advance the education and general wellbeing of children with adequate intelligence who have learning disabilities arising from perceptual, conceptual or subtle coordinative problems, sometimes accompanied by behaviour difficulties'.)

> Closer Look
> P.O. Box 1492
> Washington D C 20013

(An information centre for parents of handicapped children, Closer Look has five other branches and takes in a wider range of children.)

> *The Directory for Exceptional Children* published by Porter, Sargent Publishers Inc.
> 11 Beacon Street
> Boston
> Mass 02108

(The Directory lists many private establishments for the learning disabled. The description of each school/facility generally quotes the I Q range for children eligible for acceptance, gives the usual length of treatment (anything from four months to six years) and states whether the establishment is 'private', 'inc. no profit', which means that it is a non-profit-making establishment, or 'no fee state aid', which means that it is publicly funded and parents are charged no fees. This very comprehensive compendium repays careful reading. It will give you very good guidance about what additional questions should be asked of any establishment being directly approached.)

Australia

Responsibility for education is divided between the central Commonwealth government and state governments. The former maintains universities, initiates, coordinates and guides policy, and provides supplementary finance. The states, each through its elected Minister for Education, are responsible for primary, secondary, technical and further education. School attendance regulations vary from one state to another, but while all children start at the age of six, they continue until they are either fifteen or sixteen. However, pre-school classes for children aged five are much used, with attendance varying from two to three hours daily, two to five days a week. In 1981, twenty-three per cent of all children were attending non-government schools, mainly denominational ones, and the number is rising.

Most states have a central curriculum unit which provides general guidelines on course planning, but schools are left with a considerable

225

degree of autonomy. Parents' associations are common, with some parent representation on school councils and boards.

Special education is provided by state governments. In all states, and especially in New South Wales, Queensland and Victoria, parents have formed voluntary organizations – such as the Crippled Children's Society, the Spastic Welfare Association and the Slow Learning Children's Group – to establish additional schools for their children with special needs. State education authorities cooperate with these groups. The Commonwealth government, through the Government Schools Commission, makes funds available to state education departments specifically for upgrading special educational facilities. Some grants for the same purpose are available to non-government schools. Provision varies from one state to another, but the general tendency is for children to be educated in the most 'ordinary' situation possible, and for a range of options to be made available. These options are:

1. remedial help from the regular teacher in the normal classroom;

2. support teachers attached to ordinary schools, helping children and regular teachers in the normal classroom;

3. support teachers travelling from their home-base school to help in other, normal schools;

4. part-time attendance at a special class attached to a normal school (in Queensland, for instance, thirty-seven primary schools have a special class attached to them);

5. full-time attendance at a special class attached to a normal school;

6. attendance at a special school.

School-based special/remedial services have led to an increasing number of children with disabilities being supported in ordinary schools. 'Opportunity classes' in New South Wales help children who are mildly handicapped intellectually, have severe reading problems, and, occasionally, the 'gifted'.

For the specialist teacher, Australia is remarkable for the wealth and quality of research into reading and related subjects carried out at several universities, colleges of advanced education, and in schools.

ADDRESSES
Commonwealth Schools Commission
MLC Tower Woden

P.O. Box 34
Woden A C T 2606

National Council of Independent Schools
P.O. Box 279
Woden A C T 2606

(Parents may consult either of the above, or the local branch of a specialist group such as the Crippled Children's Society.)

The first source of information and help will be the appropriate State Education Authority, listed below:

New South Wales State Office
Department of Education
G.P.O. Box 596
Haymarket
New South Wales 2001

Victoria State Office
Department of Education
450 St Kilda Road
Melbourne
Victoria 3004

South Australia State Office
Department of Education
Red Cross House
228 North Terrace
Adelaide 5000

Queensland State Office
Department of Education
G.P.O. 586
Brisbane
Queensland 4001

Tasmania State Office
Department of Education
G.P.O. 1349 N
Hobart
Tasmania 7001

Australian Capital Territory Office
P.O. Box 1573
Canberra City, A C T 2601

Northern Territory Office
Department of Education
P.O. Box 476
Darwin
Northern Territory 5794

Western Australia State Office
Department of Education
P.O. Box 6032
Hay Street East
Perth
Western Australia 6000

Canada

226 The twelve provincial governments are the main providers of education. The federal government is responsible directly for the education of Indians, Inuit, the armed forces and their dependants; it also provides extensive financial assistance to the provincial departments of education.

Arrangements vary from one province to another in many important particulars, such as the age for compulsory entry into school and for school-leaving, the division into elementary and secondary schooling, policy on tax support for 'separate schools' (schools run by religious groups), and policy on independent schools (which are attended by four per cent of all schoolchildren). And in the province of Quebec the first language is French. It is therefore absolutely essential to consult the provincial department of education; each is headed by an elected minister and administered by a deputy minister who is an appointed public servant.

Provision for children with special needs also varies from province to province. In some it includes enriched and accelerated programmes for the academically gifted. Nationally, something between five and ten per cent of all pupils are considered to come within the category of handicapped, but again the definition varies. Schools for the handicapped are financed and administered both directly by individual provinces and by interprovincial agreement. In general the aim is to integrate as many handicapped pupils as possible into their neighbourhood schools. If a special class is indicated, it too should be integrated into the setting of the local schools.

In practice, provision follows the usual gradations:

1. The regular classroom teacher deals with problems, perhaps after consultation with colleagues on the staff.

2. Regular classroom teaching is supplemented with teaching by other regular staff.

3. Special resources are brought in from a resource centre.

4. After diagnosis by a specialist or specialists, a prescriptive service is provided on regular school premises (Quebec and Saskatchewan emphasize the value of early diagnosis).

5. Placement in a special class, part-time or full-time, is arranged.

6. Placement in a special school is arranged.

Throughout Canada, parents are acknowledged and supported as the most important contributors in home programmes, and in orientation and socialization centres.

Specialist teachers will be interested in the Ontario educational TV programmes. These are carried by TELIDON, a two-way TV computer communication system with a rapidly expanding data base for educational materials.

ADDRESSES
The Hospital for Sick Children
Room 1218
555 University Avenue
Toronto, Ontario M5G 1X8

(The hospital is excellent for diagnosis generally and has a particularly helpful booklet: *The Premature Infant: A Handbook for Parents*.)

Canadian Association of Speech, Language Pathologists and Audiologists
Suite 311
44 Eglinton Avenue West
Toronto

Learning Disabilities Association of Canada
6 Kildare House
Suite 200
323 Chapel Street
Ottawa
Ontario K1N 7Z2

(The Association is interested in learning disabilities resulting from minimal brain dysfunction. The children may show any or all of the following: disturbances of conceptualization, integration, coordination, auditory perception, or visual perception.)

Federation of Independent Schools of Canada
11013 38th Street
Edmonton
Alberta T5W 2E7

Canadian Teachers' Federation
110 Argyle Avenue
Ottawa
Ontario K2P 1B4

CANADIAN EDUCATIONAL AUTHORITIES

Alberta

Department of Education
Devonian Building
11160 Jasper Avenue
Edmonton
Alberta T5K 0L2

British Columbia

Ministry of Education
Parliament Buildings
Victoria
British Columbia V8V 1X4

Manitoba

Department of Education
Room 506
1181 Portage Avenue
Winnipeg
Manitoba R3G 0T3

New Brunswick

Department of Education
P.O. Box 6000
Fredericton
New Brunswick E3B 5H1

Newfoundland and Labrador
Department of Education
Confederation Building
Box 4750
St John's
Newfoundland A1C 5T7

Northwest Territories

Department of Education
Yellowknife
Northwest Territories X1A 2L9

Nova Scotia

Department of Education
Box 578
Trade Mart
Halifax
Nova Scotia B3J 2S9

Ontario

Ministry of Education
Communication Services Branch
Mowat Block
Queen's Park
Toronto
Ontario M7A 1L2

Ministry of Colleges and Universities
Information Branch
Mowat Block
Queen's Park
Toronto
Ontario M7A 1B8

Prince Edward Island

Department of Education
Box 2000
Charlottetown
Prince Edward Island C1A 7N8

Quebec

Department of Education
Building G, 16th Floor
Government Buildings
Quebec
P.Q. G1R 5A5

Saskatchewan

Department of Education
2220 College Avenue
Regina
Saskatchewan S4P 3V7

Department of Continuing Education
Hurnford House
1855 Victoria Avenue
Regina
Saskatchewan S4P 3V5

Yukon

Department of Education
P.O. Box 2703
Whitehorse
Yukon Territory Y1A 2C6

South Africa

227 Education for all children is bilingual (black pupils must also study their own vernacular). In schools where English is the first language, Afrikaans is a compulsory subject. School is compulsory from rising seven to sixteen plus, divided into five primary and five secondary standards. There are two voluntary but much used sub-standards, to which the earliest entry is at the age of five years and six months. Each standard demands the attainment of a definite level of development by the pupil, involving intellectual, social and emotional factors as well as accumulation of knowledge.

For children who underachieve in relation to their scholastic potential, help is available at three levels:

1. Didactic aid (for children whose underachievement is caused

by deprivation, extensive absences from school, poor teaching or un-sympathetic handling) aims to eliminate the pupil's backlog. It takes place in the classroom, is provided by his regular teachers (after consultation with colleagues on the regular staff) and is structured to the individual child's needs. Inevitably much of it amounts to compensatory education.

2. Remedial education for specifically learning-impaired children (for instance, by inadequate concentration or sensory deficits) covers particular skills, like reading, spelling, writing or arithmetic, or particular content subjects, for example science. These children are withdrawn from regular classes for remedial tuition on a sessional basis, with the proviso that they should be as little removed from the mainstream as possible. Each child has an individualized remedial programme which prescribes, logically and systematically, the goals, content and activities of the remedial help by which his educational needs will be met.

3. Special education is provided in special schools for the handicapped (the blind, the partially sighted, the deaf, the hard of hearing, the epileptic, the cerebral-palsied, the autistic and the otherwise physically handicapped) and in some classes for the educationally mentally handicapped, these classes being attached to ordinary schools.

The School Psychological and Guidance Service, through its circuit school psychologists, is responsible for the identification of all learning-impaired children. The value of early diagnosis is emphasized. The school psychologist, who in some schools is responsible for remedial education, always has to decide whether a child referred to him should receive didactic or remedial help, or possibly special education. In the last case he can set in train further assessment procedures which may require help from medical and other specialists. Parental agreement is of course required. The school psychologist can also refer a child with serious behavioural, study, personality or emotional problems to a school clinic. Remedial teachers attached to school clinics may also visit schools in the vicinity.

The guidance component of the School Psychological Service operates in the context of differentiated education: secondary education is provided by separate academic, technical and commercial schools, and (since 1982) by twelve comprehensive schools. To quote the *South Africa Yearbook*:

Act 39 of 1967 lays down that education shall be provided in accordance with the ability, aptitude and interest of individual pupils and the needs of the country, and in this respect guidance shall be furnished to pupils.

The few contacts that the authors have had, through the Learning Difficulties Clinic at St Thomas' Hospital, with South African education were with English-speaking independent schools. These proved very understanding of the children's difficulties, and cooperative and efficient in implementing the remediation programmes suggested from London.

About four per cent of white children attend schools run by religious denominations or private enterprise. In Cape Province and Natal, provincial legislation allows these schools to be multi-racial.

ADDRESSES
Association of Private Schools of South Africa
Secretary: D. E. Turner
31 St David Road
Houghton 2196

(The Association works closely with the two organizations which follow.)

Catholic Education Council
P.O. Box 614
Boksburg 1460

Board of Jewish Education
P.O. Box 2942
Johannesburg 2000

DEPARTMENTS OF EDUCATION

Director of Education
P.O. Box 13
Cape Town 8000

Director of Education
Private Bag X76
Pretoria 0001

Director of Education
P.O. Box 395
Pietermaritzburg 3200

Director of Education
P.O. Box 521
Bloemfontein 9300

Director of Education
Administration of South West Africa
Administration Buildings
Windhoek 9100

Department of National Education
Private Bag X122
Pretoria 0001

Director of Education
Administration of Coloured Affairs
Private Bag X9008
Cape Town 8000

Education Branch
Department of Indian Affairs
Private Bag X4323
Durban 4000

also

Joint Matriculation Board
P.O. Box 3854
Pretoria 0001

Other countries

For other countries where education is wholly or substantially in English, consult the country's official year-book. This will contain basic information. Further questions can be put to the representative, resident in Great Britain, of the country concerned.

228

Abbreviations

ADD	attention deficit disorder
ASM	auditory sequential memory
BAS	British Ability Scales
BPVS	British Picture Vocabulary Scale
CA	chronological age
COP	Classroom Observation Procedure, for use with children aged 6+ to 7+
DORRS	Development of Reading and Related Skills, for use with older children
EEG	electroencephalogram, used to measure electrical discharges from the surface of the brain
EFA	essential fatty acids
ENT	ear, nose and throat
IQ	intelligence quotient
ITPA	Illinois Test of Psycholinguistic Abilities
LARSP	Language Acquisition and Remediation Speech Programme
MBD	minimal brain dysfunction/damage
NFER	National Foundation for Educational Research, part of Thomas Nelson, publishers
RA	reading age
RL	readability level
SDD	specific developmental dyslexia
spoken language	expressive language which includes vocabulary, syntax, articulation and intonation. (Also called oracy)
VSM	visual sequential memory
WISC-R	Wechsler Intelligence Scale for Children Revised

Index

Illustrative Index

An illustrative index of case-histories giving the complaint that brought the child to the clinic. The paragraph identifying the child's main problem is listed by title, together with its relevant page number.

FOR THE BEST IN PAPERBACKS, LOOK FOR THE

In every corner of the world, on every subject under the sun, Penguin represents quality and variety – the very best in publishing today.

For complete information about books available from Penguin – including Pelicans, Puffins, Peregrines and Penguin Classics – and how to order them, write to us at the appropriate address below. Please note that for copyright reasons the selection of books varies from country to country.

In the United Kingdom: For a complete list of books available from Penguin in the U.K., please write to *Dept E.P., Penguin Books Ltd, Harmondsworth, Middlesex, UB7 0DA*

In the United States: For a complete list of books available from Penguin in the U.S., please write to *Dept BA, Penguin, 299 Murray Hill Parkway, East Rutherford, New Jersey 07073*

In Canada: For a complete list of books available from Penguin in Canada, please write to *Penguin Books Canada Ltd, 2801 John Street, Markham, Ontario L3R 1B4*

In Australia: For a complete list of books available from Penguin in Australia, please write to the *Marketing Department, Penguin Books Australia Ltd, P.O. Box 257, Ringwood, Victoria 3134*

In New Zealand: For a complete list of books available from Penguin in New Zealand, please write to the *Marketing Department, Penguin Books (NZ) Ltd, Private Bag, Takapuna, Auckland 9*

In India: For a complete list of books available from Penguin, please write to *Penguin Overseas Ltd, 706 Eros Apartments, 56 Nehru Place, New Delhi, 110019*

In Holland: For a complete list of books available from Penguin in Holland, please write to *Penguin Books Nederland B.V., Postbus 195, NL–1380AD Weesp, Netherlands*

In Germany: For a complete list of books available from Penguin, please write to *Penguin Books Ltd, Friedrichstrasse 10 – 12, D–6000 Frankfurt Main 1, Federal Republic of Germany*

In Spain: For a complete list of books available from Penguin in Spain, please write to *Longman Penguin España, Calle San Nicolas 15, E–28013 Madrid, Spain*

FOR THE BEST IN PAPERBACKS, LOOK FOR THE 🐧

A CHOICE OF PENGUINS AND PELICANS

Metamagical Themas Douglas R. Hofstadter

A new mind-bending bestseller by the author of *Gödel, Escher, Bach*.

The Body Anthony Smith

A completely updated edition of the well-known book by the author of *The Mind*. The clear and comprehensive text deals with everything from sex to the skeleton, sleep to the senses.

Why Big Fierce Animals are Rare Paul Colinvaux

'A vivid picture of how the natural world works' – *Nature*

How to Lie with Statistics Darrell Huff

A classic introduction to the ways statistics can be used to prove *anything*, the book is both informative and 'wildly funny' – *Evening News*

The Penguin Dictionary of Computers Anthony Chandor and others

An invaluable glossary of over 300 words, from 'aberration' to 'zoom' by way of 'crippled lead-frog tests' and 'output bus drivers'.

The Cosmic Code Heinz R. Pagels

Tracing the historical development of quantum physics, the author describes the baffling and seemingly lawless world of leptons, hadrons, gluons and quarks and provides a lucid and exciting guide for the layman to the world of infinitesimal particles.